MONOGRAPH NUMBER TWENTY NINE

THE ISSUE OF EQUALITY: EUROPEAN PERCEPTIONS OF EMPLOYMENT FOR DISABLED PERSONS

by
Harlan Hahn, Ph.D.

**Department of Political Science
University of Southern California**

International Exchange of Experts and Information in Rehabilitation
World Rehabilitation Fund, Inc.
400 East 34th Street
New York, New York 10016

This investigation was supported in part by the World Rehabilitation Fund under a grant (no. G00 8103982) from the National Institute of Handicapped Research, U.S. Department of Education, Washington, DC 20201.

ISBN #939986-41-8

TABLE OF CONTENTS

FOREWORD

The WRF under a three-year grant from the National Institute of Handicapped Research has the privilege and obligation to "import" knowledge from other countries in order to stimulate new ways of thinking and doing in the field of rehabilitation in the U.S. A glance at the back pages of this book will indicate that over the past five years WRF has published twenty-nine monographs through the International Exchange of Expets and Information in Rehabilitation project. In addition seventy-three fellowships have been awarded to *U.S.* rehabilitation experts to study abroad and then to disseminate and develop further in the U.S. ideas regarding practices, programs, policies and research in rehabilitation which were studied abroad. NIHR/OSERS priorities have been used as guidelines for selection of monograph topics and fellowship studies.

In addition to preparing fellowship reports, IEEIR fellows make use of the information gained abroad in their professional practice and in dissemination efforts and activities. Usually monographs are prepared by foreign experts; however, on occasion WRF asks an IEEIR fellow to prepare a monograph for the series. Such is the case with Harlan Hahn. Dr. Hahn had been concerned with policy issues regarding equality in employment for persons with disabilities for a long time, so that his fellowship study-visit was a natural extension of one of his major concerns. The monograph is a further extension of that interest. It is an interesting side-note to know that Dr. Hahn, as a professor of political science studied rehabilitation counseling in the Master's program at California State University under Dr. Joseph Stubbins, who has also prepared a commentary on Hahn's material and Croxen's response. Dr. Hahn is a prolific writer and is currently in the process of developing a multi-disciplinary program in the study of disability and society at the University of Southern California.

Mary Croxen is affiliated with Open University in the U.K. and author of the commentary on this piece by Dr. Hahn and is involved in many academic pursuits on behalf of people with disabilities world-wide, including chairing a committee on employment of the disabled for the European Economic Council. Her critique here of Hahn's work is strong indeed, and we are aware of the difficulty she had in preparing her remarks. We trust that Hahn's, Croxen's and Stubbins' pieces will be grist for the rehabilitation mill.

Diane Woods
Project Director
International Exchange of Experts
and Information in Rehabilitation

SECTION ONE: INTRODUCTION

Recently, both in Europe and in the United States, important new perspectives have emerged concerning the employment of persons with disabilities. While innovations in the field of vocational rehabilitation obviously have stimulated fresh approaches to this issue, perhaps even more significant are the changes which have been promoted by disabled people themselves. From a group which had traditionally been regarded as passive recipients of health care and other services, disabled citizens in the nineteen-seventies began to assume an increasingly prominent role in the social and political life of many countries. In American rehabilitation, the potential influence of this trend prompted Adams (1976) to describe this period as "the age of the consumer." Subsequently, the United Nations was inspired by these developments to proclaim first a year and later a decade as the special era of disabled persons.

The growth of the international social and political movement of disabled individuals has far-reaching implications for rehabilitation professionals and for the nondisabled community. In the past, citizens with disabilities have been encouraged to accept a subservient status in most societies both by their subordinate role in medical and rehabilitation programs and by other prevalent problems which plague disadvantaged groups such as presumptions of biological inferiority, inadequate educational opportunities, persistent unemployment, welfare dependency, endemic poverty, and a vast system of attitudinal and behavioral barriers to fulfillment of the rights of citizenship. Perhaps most fundamentally, their strength has been diminished by their understandable reluctance to organize and mobilize politically around that aspect of themselves—their disabilities—which is most negatively stigmatized by the rest of society. Deprived of the chance to form a cohesive political force through frequent interaction with each other, disabled people have been neglected or ignored when major legislative and administrative decisions were made about their prospects of securing employment and attaining other crucial objectives. As a result, historical patterns in the study of vocational rehabilitation or in the development of employment policy for disabled persons often failed to reflect the needs and desires of this segment of the population.

Gradually, however, a growing proportion of the disabled population is becoming aware of a new understanding of the nature and meaning of physical disability. In many areas of the world, individuals with disabilities are meeting to discuss their common experiences and to identify the distinctive values which they share. Even more importantly, some are beginning to comprehend disability as a potential source of pride and dignity instead of shame. Despite the numerous obstacles which they have encountered, disabled persons have displayed a mental and emotional strength which is evidence not only of the resilience of the human spirit but also of the relative unimportance of the emphasis on physical standards in modern civilization. Many have begun to perceive their problems as resulting from the policies adopted by a predominantly nondisabled society rather than from other causes.

The agenda proposed by the political movement of disabled persons is extensive. Many disabled activists in the United States and Europe are seeking not only a major improvement in the social and economic status of this segment of the population but also a massive restructuring of the built environment and sweeping changes in public attitudes and behavior. Moreover, they are phrasing their arguments in terms of basic values such as equality and freedom which are widely respected in democratic nations. Increasing numbers of disabled persons are beginning to realize that the concept of liberty is severely restricted in a country in which citizens are guaranteed international travel rights but prevented by architectural barriers or inhospitable environments from moving freely in their own neighborhoods and communities. Similarly, equality may have relatively little meaning to disabled individuals who are prohibited by unattainable physical requirements from enjoying the same rights and privileges that are available to the nondisabled. These principles have important implications for employment as well as for other activities. The refusal to hire a worker because of the functional limitations of a disability, for example, is not yet widely accepted as a denial of equal rights; but various understandings of the concept of equality permit this interpretation. Since the major differences between European and American approaches to the hiring of disabled workers seem to reflect divergent understandings of the principle of equality, this study focuses on a comparative examination of employment policies utilizing values and perspectives derived from the political movement of citizens with disabilities.

The organization of the monograph is divided into five sections.

In the **second section**, an attempt is made to grapple with the crucial problem of the definition of disability. After reviewing three different definitions based on medical, economic, and socio-political perspectives, the problems of disabled persons as a minority group in modern society are examined. Concepts of visibility and permanence are explored as a basis for developing a disability continuum which could be used as an operational measure of a sociopolitical definition. The final portion of this section discusses the implications of the three definitions for the study of disability.

Section three focuses on European and American understandings of the concept of equality which appears to offer an important theoretical vantage point for the analysis of employment policies affecting people with disabilities. In addition, a description is provided of the principal methods used in this research on European perceptions regarding the issue of employment.

In **section four**, an effort is made, insofar as possible, to allow the respondents in this study to speak for themselves. Opinions and assessments are presented concerning a wide range of problems affecting the employment of persons with disabilities. Portions of this discussion, however, also reflect an attempt to probe some of the values contained in European policies.

The final section evaluates some of the policy implications of this study. Particular attention is devoted to the potential applicability of the European experience to the theory and practice of rehabilitation in the United States.

Much of the impetus for the increasing effort by disabled persons to exert an impact on the formulation of employment and other policies also can be traced to a significant shift in the definition of disability (Hahn, 1982). Both the nature of research and policy recommendations that result in the development of programs are strongly influenced by conceptual orientations which shape investigations of the problem. In the study of disability, scientists and service-delivery personnel are at the brink of a revolutionary change in paradigms which is inextricably related to the social and political movement of people with disabilities (DeJong, 1983). Since this transition is certain to alter the theory as well as the practice of rehabilitation, a careful delineation of definitional issues seems indispensible to comparative analysis.

Medical, Economic, and Socio-Political Definitions of Disability

Perhaps the most traditional and popular definitions reflects a *medical* concept which tends to equate disability with functional impairment. From this perspective, a disability is viewed primarily as an organic defect or deficiency which is located exclusively within the individual. Principal attention is devoted to the clinical task of expanding a disabled patient's physical capacities to the maximum extent possible, and little or no consideration is given to the potential of improving personal circumstances through changes in laws or social policy. This approach to disability is based on a medical model which Osmond and Siegler (1979) have defined as consisting of Aesculepian authority, or the uniquely benevolent guidance of a physician, and of Parson's concept of the ''sick role'' that exempts individuals from usual social roles provided that they surrender to the direction of medical personnel and commit themselves solely to the ultimate goal of complete recovery. Since the paramount objective is a restoration of physical functioning, the medical definition of disability encompasses most of the difficulties of a theoretical framework which is designed primarily for acute rather than chronic conditions. Despite their best efforts, many of the problems of disability cannot be ameliorated only through heroic intervention by skilled practitioners in the health sciences or related disciplines. As a result, there appears to be an increasing interest in the development of alternative models which might augment or supplement the benefits provided by a medical approach to disability.

Medical perspectives also are influenced by a dominant emphasis on etiology, or the study of the causes of health conditions. To many disabled individuals, the question of causation seems secondary to the effects produced not only by physical impairments but also by the perceptions which disability may elicit from others. Moreover, overwhelming interest in research on the causes of disablement might appear to support pervasive cultural values which suggest that the elimination or eradication of disability is the ultimate solution to the problem. (Such values may be deeply disturbing to persons who cannot divest themselves of their disabilities.) Despite impressive scientific progress, demographic projections indicate that the proportion of disabled persons in the population is likely to grow rather than to decline in the future. In fact, medical research has been a major determinant of this trend by promoting increased longevity, which is directly associated with the prevalence of disability, and by developing advanced technologies which have permitted many people who might otherwise have died to survive with severe disabilities.

Perhaps one of the most important consequences of the stress on etiology in the medical approach, however, has resulted from the tendency to view disability primarily within the context of separate diagnostic categories. People with cerebral palsy, spinal-cord injuries, hearing or visual impairments, and a host of other conditions considered disabilities are perceived as having different problems. Little effort is made to identify the social and economic disadvantages, or even the visible impairments, which disabled persons may share; and separate organizations have been formed to represent or to assist individuals in each diagnostic classification. Hence, the medical model has fostered a type of fragmentation which has inhibited the formation of alliances or coalitions and the development of the disability community as a unified social, economic, and political force in society.

A second major definition of disability embodies an *economic* orientation which focuses on vocational limitations. According to Berkowitz, Johnson, and Murphy (1976), for example, a disability is "a health-related inability or limitation on the amount or kind of work that an individual can perform." Unlike the medical perspective which was derived from concepts and assumptions of the health sciences, the economic definition did not seem to emerge from any specific academic discipline. Incorporated first in public policy, the concept of work disability became the basis for programs in vocational training and guidance which were designed principally to promote the reintegration of disabled persons into the labor force. In the United States, the field of rehabilitation counseling developed as one of the major responses to these policy directives. Although there does not appear to be an exact equivalent to this profession in Europe (Carnes, 1979), many public and private agencies in those countries provide similar services in occupational evaluation and placement for disabled individuals. Thus, programs to alleviate the problems of a disability have tended to revolve about economic issues.

Perhaps a major difficulty permeating the economic definition of disability has resulted from its tendency to incorporate the assumptions of an economy based on manual labor rather than on the delivery of personal services or on sophisticated technology. At a relatively early stage of industrialization, when primary emphasis was placed on physical strength and agility, functional requirements which prevented disabled workers from gaining many types of jobs might have seemed plausible or even necessary. As conditions change in economically developed nations, as greater stress is focused on emotional and mental rather than physical skills, and as additional information is acquired about modifications of the occupational environment and the work site, the relationship between disability and work seems to become increasingly tenuous. In fact, there appear to be no more reasons for assuming that a disability would preclude an individual from entering various types of occupations than for assuming that a job could be altered to fit the needs and talents of a disabled employee.

Economic perspectives generally have tended to identify disability as a characteristic which resides within the individual rather than in the environment. Most rehabilitation programs are founded on a clinical model that regards disability as synonymous with occupational as well as functional restrictions which can be remedied through proper counseling, testing, training, and placement on a one-to-one basis (Stubbins, 1982). Consequently, medical and economic approaches to disability are not fundamentally incompatible, and professions associated with these two orientations have seemed to dominate discussion of the issue.

Gradually, however, increasing research began to reveal a close association between work disability and broader environmental influences such as the economic climate of a nation. During World War II in the United States, for example, disabled workers and women were welcomed by employers who needed their skills; physical requirements for jobs were waived, only to be reimposed when nondisabled veterans returned to the labor force. Similarly, Brehm, Howard, and Nagi (1980) discovered that applications for—and approval of—disability benefits increased in regions of the country which were experiencing economic recessions and declined in areas which were enjoying relative prosperity. Such findings clearly demonstrate that efforts to discover the meaning of disability must probe deeply into the economic and social structure rather than reflecting an exclusive on the attributes of an individual. Unfortunately, however, since existing surveys of disability are based solely on functional or economic definitions, useful statistics are almost impossible to obtain. Many disabled people who are productive members of the labor force undoubtedly are excluded from the concept of work disability.

Conversely, of course, perhaps the major weakness of the economic definition of disability is its undimensional character. A disability has an impact on all facets of life; its effects are not confined to the world of work. Although the field of rehabilitation has sought to encompass many of these issues through a study of the psychosocial aspects of disability, approaches which are oriented primarily toward economic or vocational considerations may fail to comprehend the multifaceted nature of the problems confronting disabled persons.

Increasingly, during the nineteen-seventies, a new approach, which has been termed a *socio-political* definition of disability, began to develop

(Hahn, 1982). This concept does not view disability as a trait which can be found solely within an individual. On the contrary, disability is regarded as a product of the interaction between the individual and the environment. From this perspective, the problems associated with disability are not the result of personal limitations; instead, they are primarily the consequences of a disabling environment. This orientation recognizes that most of the difficulties encountered by disabled people are external rather than internal. As a result, the theoretical foundations of the socio-political definition of disability are shifted from the clinical model of the health sciences, and even areas such as psychology and education which have been traditionally aligned with rehabilitation, to social science disciplines such as sociology and political science that facilitate the study of environmental as well as individual characteristics.

The Minority Group Perspective

Perhaps the most important insight which has emerged from the socio-political perspective is the realization that citizens with disabilities comprise a minority group in every nation of the world. This assessment, which is gaining increased acceptance among government officials and researchers, can be demonstrated both by objective indicators and by crucial theoretical considerations which have usually been neglected in prior studies. While there appears to be growing agreement that disabled persons are a minority (Saffilios-Rothschild, 1970; Gliedman and Roth, 1979; Eisenberg, Griggins, and Duvall, 1982), the concept has not yet been effectively incorporated into the major fields concerned with disability such as rehabilitation and medicine.

Even though the uses of available data are significantly diminished by their exclusive reliance on functional or vocational definitions of disability, numerous surveys reveal that disabled persons are the victims of greater social, economic, and political deprivation than other groups which are commonly regarded as minorities. In the United States, for example, existing evidence demonstrates that, in comparison with ethnic or racial minorities, disabled citizens have the highest rates of unemployment and welfare dependency as well as the largest proportion of persons below the poverty line (Bowe, 1978). Most disabled individuals have been taught in separate schools, subjected to extensive institutionalization, and segregated in transportation, housing, and other areas of everyday life. Even the features of the built environment and the ubiquitous network of architectural barriers that permeates society can be viewed as bars which prevent persons from exercising the rights of citizenship and which prohibit the integration of disabled and nondisabled segments of the population. In fact, disabled people have been forced to accommodate to a system of segregation that is more widespread and restrictive than even the most rigid laws of racial or ethnic separation directed at other minorities. Such facts clearly document the minority status of citizens with disabilities because they disclose the discriminatory *effects* of overt or covert policies that have compelled disabled persons to assume a subordinate role in society. Much more difficult, however, is the effort to discover the *sources* of this form of prejudice and segregation.

While the fundamental reasons for discrimination against persons with disabilities must remain a subject of conjecture, the definition grounded on socio-political considerations appears to be compatible with several interpretations which have important implications for future research. Finkelstein (1980), for example, has suggested that attitudes about disability may be shaped by pervasive economic and social systems and especially by the difficulty of fitting disabled people into organized modes of production developed in the process of industrialization. Clearly economic trends for several centuries have promoted standardized patterns of manufacturing and consumption that impose physical requirements which are intrinsically incompatible with the concept of individuation, or a system designed to satisfy the interests and needs of all persons including those with disabilities. Yet, prejudice toward disabled people also has been attributed to a combination of ''existential and esthetic anxiety'' among the nondisabled (Hahn, 1983). Many persons may attempt to avoid and to isolate disabled individuals not only because they are viewed as alien and different but also because the specter of disability is regarded as a serious threat to their lifestyles and their bodily integrity. These theories seem to connote different solutions to the problems encountered by citizens with disabilities. Whereas the former appears to imply that the eradication of discrimination against disabled persons can only be accomplished through massive changes in economic organization and philosophy, the latter seems to propose that this goal might be achieved through policies designed to combat bias and segregation. In either event, the recognition that disabled citizens often become the objects of discrimination offers a strong refutation to the popular view of disability simply as a personal misfortune. The difficulties confronting people with disabilities do not emanate from sources which can be found within the individual. Instead, they are primarily the products of social, economic, and political forces located in the environment which envelopes disabled persons.

Many questions, however, remain unanswered. In view of the vast sympathy which is displayed toward individuals with disabilities, what is the basis for this pattern of discrimination? How can rehabilitation professionals in America or in other countries attempt to combat it?

Although research based on the socio-political approach has not yet developed sufficiently to furnish a definitive answer to these questions, some speculation can be offered which might provide direction for further investigations and contribute to a clarification of the definition of disability. Perhaps one of the most obvious and yet one of the most neglected aspects of disability is the extent to which it represents a departure or deviation from dominant standards of bodily appearance or behavior. Among the many attributes that disabled persons have in common with other minority groups, probably none are more salient or significant than the physical characteristics which set them off from the majority. Along with visible physical traits which reflect race or ethnicity, gender, and age, therefore, disabilities often become cues which trigger aversive or prejudicial reactions from others. Fundamentally, while disabled citizens share many social, economic, and political problems with all minorities, perhaps their basic similarity is the presence of characteristics which permit them to become the objects of differentiation and discrimination. Without these identifiable physical differences, disabled persons could not be subjected to the same processes of stereotyping, stigmatizing, bias, prejudice, discrimination, and segregation that plague every minority group. Moreover, when such traits are coupled with adverse social labeling, the effects of discrimination are compounded.

Concepts of Visibility and Permanency

From this perspective, two of the most important dimensions of the characteristics of disabled persons—and of other minorities—are permanence and visibility. Unlike most similar groups, membership in the disabled minority usually is not genetically determined. Some highly stigmatized disabilities such as epilepsy are episodic rather than continuous. Yet, whether a disability occurs in childhood, adolescence, or later in life, few persons in this minority can anticipate either a complete cure or total concealment as a solution to the problems which they encounter. The distinction between temporary and enduring personal attributes seems crucial, and perhaps even more critical than the age of onset, because it is directly related to the fundamental issue of identity. In the past, many persons, deprived of positive references which would enable them to identify their physical differences as beautiful or as sources of dignity and pride, have attempted to disguise or ignore their disabilities in the hope of gaining greater acceptance by the nondisabled majority. But disabilities do not have the qualities of a chameleon, and "passing" is a luxury which can be indulged only at great psychological peril. Eventually, numerous individuals have found it necessary to incorporate a disability into their own self-concepts and to recognize it as a target of discrimination rather than as an object of embarrassment or humiliation. Permanence may be essential to the development of identification and, as such, indispensible to the definition of disability.

Perhaps an even more significant component of an enhanced understanding of the meaning of disability, however, is the element of visibility. Clearly, disabilities vary in the extent to which they are recognizable or perceptible to other people. While some may be immediately obvious, others might become apparent only through careful observation, close scrutiny, or intimate knowledge of an individual. Many disabilities might be noticed when a person is motionless, but others may not be disclosed until the individual engages in a variety of physical or social activities. People also may differ in their capacities to detect the presence of a disability. Yet, if disabilities are primarily characteristics that evoke aversion or prejudicial responses from others, it should be possible to develop a disability continuum ranging from the most visible, which may be expected to elicit intense stigmatizing, to the least visible, which seldom becomes the targets of segregation or discrimination:

Figure 1—The Disability Continuum

Most Visible   **Least Visible**
/ ______/ ______/ ______/ ______/ ______/ ______/ ______/ ______/ ______/
Most Discrimination   **Least Discrimination**

Moreover, this conceptualization would permit the delineation of "thresholds" along the continuum, representing the amount of discrimination directed at persons with disabilities of differing degrees of visibility. Thus, individuals with disabilities which deviate greatly from conventional images of the human form may be exposed to the most extreme forms of stereotyping and stigmatizing, followed by people with less perceptible differences, and finally by those whose disabilities may become evident only through careful inspection. The continuum is founded on the assumption that observable differences which allow differentiation between the members of minority groups and the dominant majority are the essential bases for prejudice and segregation. It permits an examination of the association between discrimination and the visibility of physical characteristics such as a disability. As further information is gathered, additional dimensions might be added to provide a more comprehensive or parsimonious explanation of discrimination against disabled persons. However, as an intitial attempt to incorporate the concepts of visibility and permanence into the definition of disability, this continuum seems to offer the hope of gaining an improved understanding of the problems which confront disabled citizens in employment as sell as other areas of life.

Unfortunately, existing data, which are based exclusively on functional or economic definitions of disability, do not provide an opportunity to test the relationship between visibility and discrimination proposed by this continuum. Medical research on persons in various diagnostic categories seldom seeks to measure the extent to which a disability may be perceptible to others, and even the degree of impairment often is treated as secondary to etiological concerns. Similarly, studies of work disability usually make no mention of visibility, and only a few studies have attempted to examine the association between this type of disability and economic models of employment discrimination (Johnson and Lambrinos, 1983). Even though there is abundant evidence that disabilities trigger prejudicial behavior, available information does not provide an adequate basis for exploring the origins of this type of conduct.

A definition of disability that embodies the principles of visibility and permanence, however, may introduce some major changes in existing efforts to delineate the meaning of this term. Although primary emphasis is placed on physical characteristics which may trigger prejudice and discrimination, this approach does not necessarily exclude people with mental or emotional disabilities. In fact, one of the major attributes supposedly shared by persons with physical, mental, and emotional disabilities is the perception by others that they may engage in socially awkward, inappropriate, or unacceptable behavior. From this perspective, disability is solely an image in the mind of the beholder which might be projected onto other individuals whose appearance or demeanor is regarded as unconventional or intolerable. The disability continuum supersedes traditional diagnostic categories which have been created within the medical model as well as other distinctions such as physical impairments, developmental disabilities, and problems of mental or emotional health. Since all persons within these groups may display physical traits which make them targets of discrimination, their similarities as members of a common minority appear to overshadow the differences between them which have become such a salient focus of attention for the nondisabled majority. As a result, use of the concept of visibility seems to hold important promise not only for fruitful research but also for the formation of unity or social and political alliances among people with disabilities.

The application of the criterion of permanence to persons with emotional or mental disabilities, however, seems somewhat more problematic. Although such individuals often are subjected to discriminatory treatment, programs designed for this segment of the population may offer the hope of complete relief from symptoms as a solution to their problems. Thus, psychological difficulties sometimes are perceived as temporary rather than as continuing sources of identification with a disadvantaged segment of society. These considerations seem especially relevant to conditions such as alcoholism and drug abuse, increasingly regarded as medical instead of personal issues, which are viewed as disabilities in Sweden and, for some purposes, in the United States. While many persons regard efforts to combat these conditions as a continuing struggle, others do not necessarily share this perspective. Perhaps objective criteria of permanence must be combined with a subjective component. People become disabled primarily because they are treated as disabled and, through the effects of stigmatizing and discrimination, begin to recognize their status as disabled individuals. Scott (1981), for example, found that, even for a condition such as blindness which is supposedly susceptible to scientific measurement, membership in the group was determined less by the degree of vision impairment than by a process of socialization into the role of blind persons. An important defining characteristic of a disability, therefore, is the extent to which it promotes a feeling of affiliation with persons in similar circumstances. Insofar as emotional and mental problems are widely recognized as encompassing physical manifestations that permit the differentiation upon which discrimination is based, persons possessing those traits may experience a strong and enduring sense of affinity with the disabled minority.

An important advantage of a definition containing the disability continuum is its capacity to eliminate some of the confusion resulting from prior distinctions between so-called ''hidden'' disabilities and those which are instantly indentifiable by others. Many of the most prevalent forms of disability are not highly visible in most situations. Yet all might become obvious through close observation, and each can be used as a basis for discrimination. A continuum recognizes this potential for prejudicial conduct by including a series of thresholds which may indicate the degree of bias directed at persons with various types of disabilities. Similarly, the continuum transcends differences between sensory disabilities and mobility impairments. Difficulties in communication stemming from vision or hearing loss are readily noticeable in personal interactions and often produce unequal treatment in the same manner as other stigmatized disabilities. Perhaps the most crucial factor is the willingness of individuals with various types of ''hidden'' or seemingly unapparent disabilities to identify themselves as disabled persons. While people with relatively imperceptible disabilities generally may encounter less prejudice than their counterparts at the opposite end of the continuum, they are constantly exposed to the threat of discrimination in specific contexts and at certain critical junctures in their lives. As a result, a definition of disability based on visibility and permanence provides a framework for recognizing the common nature of the obstacles confronting all disabled people and for developing an enhanced awareness of the need for plans to resolve these problems.

Even more significantly, this definition offers the opportunity to include a consideration of the environment in the investigation of disability-related phenomena. Although the concepts of permanence and visibility focus attention principally on the attitudes and behavior of the nondisabled majority, other important elements of the milieu surrounding disabled people also can be examined with this approach. From a socio-political perspective, for example, configurations of the man-made environment which inhibit freedom of movement by disabled persons or which require them to engage in behaviors inconsistent with their limitations cannot be regarded merely as unfortunate or accidental. Like all other features of society, artificial barriers and social conventions having a detrimental effect on persons with disabilities are the products of implicit or explicit policies which reflect values that are widely shared among crucial segments of the population. The fact that they allegedly were not intended to foster segregation does not lessen their discriminatory impact. Moreover, these aspects of the environment reinforce prevalent public tendencies to avoid, isolate, and segregate people with dis-

16

abilities. As a result, any definition that is used as a basis for developing programs for disabled individuals must incorporate an assessment of environmental constraints which consign them to the status of second-class citizens.

A reconceptualization of disability that takes cognizance of the existence of discrimination also could save rehabilitation and health professionals from the pitfalls of the fallacy which Ryan (1971) has called "blaming the victim." Too often the difficulties of disabled persons are ascribed personality traits such as to a lack of motivation or an inability to make a successful adjustment to the limitations of a disability. These appraisals seem to assume that the disadvantages plaguing relatively powerless groups such as individuals with disabilities, are caused by their personal actions and that their status can be improved merely by emulating the behavior of dominant and influential segments of the population. Little attention is devoted to aspects of the social and economic structure or to policies and regulations which contribute to their subordinate role in society. Yet the principal source of the problems associated with disability are located outside rather than inside disabled individuals. In fact, most of the obstacles confronting disabled citizens stem from their position as members of a minority group rather than from their functional impairments or their vocational deficits. By placing an increased emphasis on environmental considerations and on the persistent issue of discrimination, this approach to the definition of disability might avoid a simplistic and erroneous assessment of the needs and aspirations of people with disabilities.

Implications of the Three Definitions

The medical, economic, and socio-political definitions of disability seem to represent separate dimensions of a multifaceted problem. But each also implies need for a different solution. In the field of employment, for example, medical and economic concepts appear to suggest that the best way to promote the hiring of disabled workers entails efforts to improve their fundamental capacities or their occupational skills, respectively. Both seem to reflect an essentially clinical orientation which focuses on individual capabilities and preparation. Both also seem to embody assumptions of biological inferiority similar to those which were once directed at racial and ethnic minorities, women, and aging persons.

By contrast, the socio-political approach indicates that the major sources of the employment difficulties confronting disabled persons are located in the environment and especially in patterns of discrimination which have traditionally denied them civil rights. From this vantage point, persistent unemployment in the disability community can be attributed primarily to stereotypes which prevent employers from recognizing the talents of disabled applicants for jobs, stigmatizing attitudes which creates worries about how disabled employees would be greeted by their co-workers, bias which yields of job requirements that bear little relation to physical or other tasks necessary to perform the work, prejudice which causes management to discount disabled job seekers without a fair evaluation of their qualifications, discrimination which is produced by a desire to avoid and to reject disabled people at work as well as in other social settings, and segregation which is reinforced by a belief that worksites cannot be modified or made accessible to disabled persons. When these practices are combined with the effects of pervasive separation in education, transportation, and other facilities that are essential to the pursuit of jobs, the frustrations induced by an inability to obtain meaningful work may become debilitating. Unlike the prescriptions offered by medical and economic perspectives, however, employment discrimination cannot be eliminated solely by individual effort. Instead, policies must be promulgated establishing legal standards to eliminate prejudice against disabled persons in the workplace and in the community. As a result, the focus of attention is shifted from hospitals, rehabilitation facilities, and similar institutions to the political process which is responsible for providing equal rights to all citizens, including those with disabilities.

Each of the three major definitions of disability has already been adopted in public policy. In the United States and in many European nations, government programs to provide employment for disabled persons through vocational rehabilitation gained increasing approval after the end of World War I. Similarly, public support for medical efforts to improve the functional capabilities of individuals with disabilities has been enacted in many countries. Moreover, during the nineteen-seventies, important ingredients of the socio-political perspective which focuses on the environment rather than the individual began to appear in statutes. Perhaps the clearest expression of this trend was contained in Section 504 of the U.S. Rehabilitation Act of 1973, which stated: "No otherwise qualified handicapped individual shall, solely by reason of his handicap, be denied benefits under or be prohibited from participating in any program receiving substantial Federal financial assistance." Although few other nations have enacted comparable civil rights legislation for people with disabilities, an anti-discrimination bill was introduced and debated in the British Parliament. In addition, numerous countries have endorsed measures to change the discriminatory effects of the social and economic environment upon disabled citizens. Perhaps most importantly, the increasing acceptance of this new approach to disability has prompted a mounting world-wide awareness among people with disabilities that the primary sources of their problems are prejudice and discrimination rather than functional impairments or vocational deficiencies. As a result, a growing international movement, based on a socio-political understanding of the nature of disability, promises to produce important future changes in laws and policies affecting the treatment of disabled persons.

Although the implications of the socio-political approach appear to be relatively sweeping, none of the three principal definitions of disability seems fundamentally incompatible with theoretical traditions in the study of this subject. One of the most widely respected prior definitions, for example, is the formulation proposed by Nagi (1979) who said that a "disability is an inability or limitation in performing the roles expected of an individual within a social environment." Perhaps the crucial difference between medical, economic, and socio-political orientations is the extent to which they might emphasize separate words or phrases in this statement. From the somewhat individualistic perspectives of medical and economic concepts, major stress seems to be placed on the "inability or limitation" and perhaps on the notion of "performance" in coping with daily life and the demands of employment. Insofar as the external influences are considered at all, the economic model tends to focus almost solely on the job environment or the world of work. Conversely, the socio-political meaning of disability ascribes primary importance not only to the "social environment," which is the source of prejudice and discrimination, but also to the idea of "roles" and "expectations." In fact, the word "expected" is probably the operative term in the definition. In context, it apparently refers to what is anticipated by others rather than to self-expectations. In many respects, people with disabilities have experienced difficulty in seeking to conform to the standards of appearance and behavior prescribed by the rest of society. Yet human beings do not exist solely for the purpose of fulfilling the expectations of others. Moreover, the roles which an individual is "expected" to play in any environment are not governed by immutable or universal laws. In fact, the only restrictions on the capacity to produce an environment compatible with the interests and needs of all people with disabilities probably are the limitations of man's imagination. Anticipations simply reflect widely occupied beliefs about how people ought to handle themselves in a social community. Perhaps increased efforts must be made to alter pervasive expectations about human traits and activities rather than to change the characteristics of disabled persons.

There is, however, an even more fundamental level at which various interpretations of the meaning of disability must be considered. As Stubbins (1982) has pointed out, the definition of disability is, in the final analysis, determined by public policy. In other words, a disability is ultimately whatever elected officials say it is. All of the criteria developed by researchers from different schools of thought in the study of disability, including functional impairments, occupational limitations, and the concepts of visibility and permanence, can only inform the content of government laws and regulations. Eventual responsibility for making critical choices between alternative definitions is vested in political decision-makers. Moreover, their decisions are not confined to technical subjects or to theoretical questions. Public leaders also have a duty to express prevalent popular understandings of an issue in the formulation of policy. Politics is, in Easton's (1971) words, "the authoritative allocation of values in society." While some of these values represent material resources, others reflect the highly intangible but deeply cherished principles upon which a country is founded. Hence, the study of disability, and of any other subject which becomes a legitimate concern of governments, cannot be divorced from the examination of values. Many such values are encapsulated in national environments that are also shaped by public policy. These environments clearly have different effects upon disabled and nondisabled segments of the population. Perhaps one of the principal tasks of research based upon a socio-political approach to disability, therefore, is the comparative examination of values implicit in the legislation of several nations. While the discussion of theoretical perspectives may contribute to the clarification of the definition of disability, its fundamental meaning must be pursued through a cross-national investigation of public policy.

SECTION THREE: EUROPEAN AND AMERICAN
CONCEPTS OF EQUALITY

Human communities seem to reflect normative expectations about the physical characteristics of their members. In most Western countries, for example, preference is accorded to persons who are young, white, and male. Individuals who possess physical traits which indicate that they belong to a different group based on age, sex, or ethnic or racial heritage not only confront severe disadvantages in their attempts to secure the rewards which a nation has to offer; but they also acquire distinct experiences by living in the environments with which they must contend. No amount of sensitivity or insight can permit outsiders to comprehend fully the lives of black people in a predominantly white world, the struggles of women within organizational structures dominated by male values and perspectives, or the lifestyles of older citizens in an overwhelmingly youth-oriented culture. As a result, many members of these groups have begun to ask other segments of the population to adapt to their needs and values rather than attempting to accommodate to the interests and requirements of the societies in which they live.

In many respects, the status of people with disabilities appears to be similar. Like other minorities, they have been the victims of prejudice and discrimination. In addition, disabled individuals have accumulated a distinctive set of life experience which may become a valuable resource for coping with an unyielding environment. Yet the stigmatizing effects of a disability often are compounded by virtually insurmountable artificial barriers. Disabled persons live in a world which was designed and constructed exclusively for the nondisabled. Frequently, disabled individuals discover that they simply cannot be there from here. For many, the difficulties which they encounter in the pursuit of major goals in life are not merely obstructions to be turned aside; they are absolute and impenetrable barricades that cannot be removed without substantial expenditures of public or private funds.

In the past, disabled people have been encouraged to circumvent such problems just as they have been urged to ''overcome'' their disabilities. But this strategy has exacted enormous costs in lost opportunities. As one person who uses a wheelchair in Sweden explained, ''The city is, for me, just a series of small oases in an otherwise vast desert. I go a few places that are familiar and where I know I won't run into trouble. But the rest of it, I just try to forget about.''

The existence of an environment which is inaccessible to large numbers of people raises some troubling but unavoidable questions about the normative assumptions which a nation might impose upon the physical capacities of its citizens. In order to pursue what most people would consider an acceptable or tolerable life, for example, should individuals be expected to walk? To run? To perform simple or routine tasks quickly? To climb a flight of steps? To see and hear clearly? To speak articulately and at a pace which is comfortable to their listeners? To eat, bathe, or dress unaided? To possess the sophistication necessary for ordinary monetary transactions? To respond in a socially appropriate manner when they are asked a question? Obviously the list of activities could be extended endlessly. Similar questions might be asked about the quality of life. What if the standards were lowered from "acceptable or tolerable" to meeting the basic necessities of life? Or raised it a satisfying and fulfilling life? The point is simple but frequently ignored. What are the minimum physical requirements which public policies define as essential for life in a society? The issue usually is cloaked in rhetoric or buried in the interstices of social service programs rather than answered in official documents. But the conclusion seems inescapable: some irreducible standard must be contained in the laws and regulations of every country in the world.

A certain mastery of the environment may be indispensible for participation in most human settlements. In the case of minorities defined solely by age, gender, and race or ethnicity, this basic condition seemingly could be satisfied by creating laws to combat discrimination without devoting extensive attention to the restructuring of the habitat. But the ultimate goals of the social and political movement of disabled people extend even beyond the development of impartial procedures to insure that the members of this minority are not treated in a stereotypical or prejudicial manner. They also include a massive rebuilding of the man-made environment. Unless sweeping efforts are made to adapt buildings, passageways, and patterns of communication to the needs and interests of individuals with disabilities, mastery of the environment may not be a feasible or realistic criteria for life in any society. Government in earlier periods of history could probably ignore this problem because few disabled citizens survived for a sufficient span of time to make them a viable segment of the population. Even fewer were equipped to endure the scorn and humiliation that accompanied their appearance in public places. As medical technology increases the longevity of disabled persons and as they acquire the self-assurance to seek expanded involvement in the life of the community, public leaders will be faced with growing dilemmas. Should the ability to master the environment be considered an essential requirement for citizenship? If so, what are the basic physical skills or abilities necessary? If not, to what extent must the environment be altered to accommodate individuals with various types of disabilities? What ought to be the purpose of these changes? To permit disabled individuals to participate in all aspects of social life or simply in those activities which are crucial to their survival? Who must make the decision?

The moral and political magnitude of these questions is enhanced when consideration is given to the enormous economic, social, psychological, and physical costs of a disability. Many disabled persons who manage to sustain themselves in an unaccommodative environment have done so through great bodily strain which may ultimately shorten their lives. They have been disproportionately subjected to the emotional anguish associated with stigma and isolation. They have been compelled to expend vast amounts of time and money on routine feats which their nondisabled counterparts find trivial and financially inconsequential. In a competitive economy which places a premium on the capacity to engage in physical activities efficiently and inexpensively, disabled employees are often at a serious disadvantage. These facts raise other disturbing questions. Are the additional expenses of a disability simply an individual responsibility, or should they be fully or partially assumed by government acting on behalf of the entire community? What about the financial burdens imposed upon disabled citizens by an inaccessible or unadapted environment? In a society in which man-made structures were planned and constructed solely for the benefit of the nondisabled majority, what criteria should be used in assessing and apportioning the costs of this policy?

The issue of disability seems to have special importance in any country which seeks, as one of its major stated objectives, to provide equal rights for its citizens. Where minorities based on age, gender, and race or ethnicity have been granted increased civil rights (which have not been achieved) through the adoption of rules which require neutral or unbiased practices in employment as well as other activities, the problems confronted by persons with disabilities seem to raise even more fundamental concerns. For this segment of the population, the elimination of prejudice and discrimination may be a necessary but not a sufficient condition for admission to full membership in society. The environmental constraints which impede the progress of the disabled minority do not consist solely of the attitudes and behavior of other people; they also include permanent structures that bear unspoken testimony to earlier preconceptions about the physical abilities required of human beings before they could be considered part of the community. Efforts to assess the segregating effects of environmental influences surrounding persons with disabilities must encompass a holistic perspective. The application of principles of equality to disabled citizens, therefore, seem to produce new and unfamiliar problems for policy-makers in many nations.

Fortunately, not all countries have approached the issue of disability or the concept of equality in a similar manner. Public policies which have been developed for the disabled segment of the population seem to reflect deeply implanted cultural values that form a critical part of the legacy of each nation. When these values are compared with broader understandings of the question of equality, they appear to provide some significant clues about methods which might be employed to resolve the difficulties faced by citizens with disabilities in many areas of the world. The purpose of this analysis is not to engage in a philosophical examination of contrasting theories of equality. Instead, the penultimate objective is the identification of specific policies and programs which might be used in a variety of cultural contexts to enhance the social, economic, and political status of disabled persons. Without an understanding to the relationship between important social values and various interpretations of equality, however, many aspects of policies adopted by other countries to promote the employment of disabled citizens might appear to be relatively meaningless.

European and American Concepts of Equality

Perhaps the most distinctive feature of the American understanding of the issue of equality is its strong commitment to the value of individualism. Lacking historical experience with feudalism and royalty, Hartz (1955) notes that the United States began and remained a country in which people believed that they were "born equal." The ability to achieve social and economic success is widely perceived as an autonomous product of personal achievement through vigorous physical, mental, and emotional exertion. This tenacious adherence to rugged or romanticized individualism is closely related to the clinical perspective which has guided medical and economic approaches to the problem of disability.

In the United States, equality has been translated into the notion of "equality of opportunity." Perhaps the classic method of illustrating the distinction between these concepts is the analogy of racers on a track. Whereas a strict interpretation of the principle of equality might require judges to recognize the undue advantages of some competitors and to intervene by assigning weights or creating different matches to equalize the contests, the idea of "equality of opportunity" simply assumes that the runners must be lined up evenly at the starting point. From the latter perspective, the outcome is solely the product of individual merit. Little consideration is given to the possibility that the very nature of the events or other environmental factors may actually determine the difference between the winners and the losers. The implications for disabled and nondisabled segments of the population appear to be relatively obvious. Since persons with disabilities are compelled to compete in an environment which resembles a labyrinth or an obstacle course rather than a smooth pathway, the opportunity to display their personal abilities by participating in a game arranged by the nondisabled reflects only a faint shadow of the hope contained in the promise of equality.

One of the most crucial tests of the American concept of "equality of opportunity" occurred during the late nineteen-sixties and early nineteen-seventies in the wake of the most intense civil rights struggles which the country had ever experienced. Statistics indicated that, during the preceding decade, black Americans and other minorities had made significant progress in the efforts to improve their social and economic position; but their achievements were outstripped by the gains of whites. The realization that the gap between these groups was not being closed prompted increased interest in a more precise measure of equality and even reparations to correct the legacy of injustices which had been foisted upon deprived and disadvantaged minorities. But this viewpoint was antithetical to the faith in individualism and the notion of a meritocracy that prevailed among white residents.

Many Americans were prepared to agree that trivial physical characteristics such as skin color should not be used as a basis for prejudging a person's value or worth, but they were not willing to acknowledge that the subordinate status of black citizens was produced by social and economic influences rather than personal attributes. They clung resolutely to the myth that relative equality could be achieved on the basis of individual merit rather than through policies designed to promote the fair representation of minorities in important positions within the structure of society. Arguments in favor of quotas floundered on deeply entrenched beliefs in individualism and ''equality of opportunity.'' Some ethnic groups, which had previously been the victims of quotas intended to exclude them from major institutions, refused to believe that this device could be used to compel the entrance of other minorities into places from which they had previously been denied access.

Perhaps most importantly, the American conviction that the principle of equality could be invoked only to insure the impartial or unbiased treatment of minorities provoked a tumultuous debate over ''reverse discrimination.'' In accordance with a view which held that the role of government should be confined to umpiring the race between individuals rather than altering the nature of the events or the design of the track, many political leaders expressed strong opposition to programs which might restrict opportunities available to the majority.

The peculiarly American response to this issue was embodied in the concept of ''affirmative action'' which reflected the nation's firm reliance on individualistic rather than structural explanations of discrimination (Livingston, 1979). This approach, which essentially required employers to establish goals in the hiring of minorities and to demonstrate reasonable progress toward the attainment of those objectives, fell far short of the explicit standards which would have been implied by a system of quotas. Disabled workers were brought within the coverage of affirmative action programs by the Rehabilitation Act of 1973 and detailed manuals have been prepared to assist employers in implementing these provisions (Zimmer, 1981). But available evidence reveals a widespread lack of compliance with the law (Bowe, 1980). Affirmative action programs have failed to reduce endemic rates of unemployment among people with disabilities, and they have not produced the results which the leaders of other minorities hoped to accomplish. Although the ultimate effects of these programs may be determined as much by litigation in the courts as by practices in personnel offices, the concept of affirmative action based on the notion of ''equality of opportunity'' has not displayed the strength or the rigor which many observers regard as necessary to combat persistent patterns of discrimination.

European approaches to the issue of equality emerged from different historical traditions and from contrasting values and expectations. In this region, the advent of industrialization was marked by titanic clashes between labor and management over the distribution of resources to social or economic classes. Governments were not confined to a passive role in these conflicts. Instead, the political process was regarded as the embodiment of important changes which were occurring in society, and public agencies often played a positive rather than a negative role in determining the allocation of benefits to various portions of the population. As a result, the concept of the welfare state, in which governments assumed responsibility for alleviating many social and economic problems, was adopted more readily in European countries than in the United States.

These trends led to the acceptance, in many nations, of certain fundamental conditions such as decent housing, adequate medical care to maintain good health, protection from the threat of systemic unemployment, and reasonable security for persons who are not working as a basic right of citizenship rather than as a privilege available only to those who can afford them. Unlike the United States which has not yet approved a comprehensive national health program, government supported medical services have been an important dimension of policy in most European countries for an extended period. Similarly, plans to support aging or retired workers and their dependents were adopted at an earlier time in Europe than in America. Numerous European efforts to assist persons who may face particular difficulties in securing employment also have become models for other nations (Reubens, 1970). Social and economic dislocations which may produce joblessness have been generally viewed as beyond the control of the individual. In addition, political leaders in Europe have tended to regard the potential productivity of the population as a form of human capital and as a crucial national resource which must be developed through investments in retraining programs and similar plans to promote the economic viability of the entire country.

Perhaps part of the dichotomy between European and American perspectives on the principle of equality also can be ascribed to different historical experiences with ethnic or racial minorities. In the United States, the struggle by these groups to achieve equal rights has been a long and prominent feature of public debate. Moreover, a written constitution and powerful legal system provided an important benchmark and a forum for assessing the extent to which these segments of the population had been treated equally.

By contrast, direct European involvement in issues of ethnic and racial equality has been relatively recent. During the prosperity of the nineteen-sixties and seventies, large numbers of unfamiliar groups such as the Turks in West Germany, the Algerians in France, and emigres from India, Pakistan, and the Caribbean who settled in Great Britain sought economic opportunities in jobs which were not being filled by indigenous labor forces. Although this pattern of immigration produced ethnic and racial strife comparable to upheavals in America, European countries lacked a constitutional tradition which might have enabled them to examine the issue in the context of persistent efforts to protect the civil rights of minority groups. As a result, even though increasing numbers of Europeans with disabilities are perceiving their problems as resulting from discrimination and segregation, the proposal of antidiscrimination measures to protect the legal rights of disabled citizens remains a foreign concept to most of Europe. Only Great Britain has given serious consideration to such a statute. Efforts to promote increased equality for disabled persons in many European nations have developed primarily from an extensive background of social welfare legislation rather than from judicial doctrines designed to guarantee individual rights. Primary attention, therefore, has been devoted to governmental programs to offset the seemingly inherent advantages enjoyed by the nondisabled by improving the social and economic position of people with disabilities.

The study of major social values embedded in policy issues has become an increasingly significant theme in cross-national research on disability and rehabilitation. Young (1984), for example, has attributed different practices in the treatment of disabled infants primarily to the dualism between the American preoccupation with individualism and the increased concern about the ''common good'' which he found in countries such as Sweden and Britain. Similarly, Purtillo (1981) revealed important discrepancies between Swedish and American atitudes in her study of concepts of liberty and justice in the context of ''humane'' health care. In addition, Stubbins (1982) disclosed variations in the emphasis on clinical attitudes in British and American rehabilitation programs. All of these investigations, by underscoring the crucial nature of the distinction between the individual and the environment, seem to reinforce the conclusion that different understandings of the sources of equality or inequality have a critical impact on people with disabilities in the United States and Europe.

European perspectives generally have assumed that primary resonsibility for overcoming egregious inequality must be assumed by governments acting on behalf of the society at large. While this orientation has evolved from an extensive intellectual tradition, perhaps the clearest expression of the sentiment can be found in platforms drafted by political parties. In Sweden, for example, a report prepared by Alva Myrdahl (quoted in Purtillo, 1981:17) for the Social Democratic party and the Confederation of Trade Unions stated: ''Equality means that where nature has created great and fundamental differences in abilities, these must not be allowed to determine the individual's chances in life, but rather that society should 'restore the balance.' These differences, in the form of physical or intellectual handicaps, can never be eliminated, but they can be reduced in a generous social climate, and one can work against their leading to social discrimination.'' Although the values contained in this position were once the subject of intense partisan conflicts, they have subsequently been endorsed by differing political persuasions throughout Europe. Notice that the statement does not fully acknowledge that disabilities are a source of discrimination; instead, it assumes that benevolent social policies can mitigate against that result.

Prevalent European definitions of equality do not necessarily attempt to achieve absolute equality or a leveling through which all citizens would be placed in a similar social and economic status. Nor do they fundamentally attempt to insure that significant minorities such as people with disabilities should be represented in important positions of influence in exact ratio to their proportions in the population. On the contrary, European perspectives appear to assume that efforts to attain relative equality entail a process of seeking equilibrium between contending interests in society. This process primarily involves groups rather than individuals. The principle of equality, as it seems to be understood by most Europeans, more closely approximates a concept of ''equal shares'' than a notion of ''equality of opportunity.'' Segments of the population are allocated resources in relation to perceived needs which might otherwise prevent them from receiving the benefits which have been defined as basic rights of a citizen such as good health and a decent standard of living. Moreover, public policy is regarded as the principal means of compensating for the intrinsic and unjustifiable disadvantages imposed upon certain portions of the national community. Major emphasis is placed on a collective approach to the solution of social problems which must be undertaken by governments rather than by private citizens. Perhaps most importantly, European countries tend to focus on societal responsibility rather than individual effort in pursuit of the goal of increased equality.

Althouth the development of employment and other policies concerning disabled persons in Europe was not directly motivated by a constant quest for equality, important implications regarding this concept can be derived from an examination of values implicit in these laws and programs. In a process that seemed to parallel the etiological concerns of the medical model, much early legislation appeared to reflect major stress on the causes of disability. Thus, even among those with similar functional impairments or vocational problems, soldiers disabled in a war were treated differently than citizens disabled by a disease, laborers disabled by industrial accidents were considered in a different manner than motorists who became disabled in automobile accidents, etc. Furthermore, these disability classifications tended to display a similar pattern not only in Europe but also in the United States and other advanced industrialized nations: disabled veterans usually received the first and the most generous benefits, followed by industrially injured workers, and then by disabled civilians (Smith and Gebert, 1981). In past, this progression may have reflected the desire of political leaders to reward citizens who were compelled to make sacrifices by serving the interests of the state in military actions or in the promotion of economic development. In any event, the differential treatment of persons who acquired their disabilities in various circumstances may have introduced an initial element of inequality to policy on this subject, but the apparent inconsistencies of this approach seemed to promote an expansion of benefits to broader segments of the disability community in Europe.

The history of disability policy in Europe and the United States can be traced to the years after World War I when the return of vast numbers of ex-servicemen prompted governments to enact legislation establishing rehabilitation programs and other provisions for the reintegration of disabled veterans into the labor force. The first laws mandating the employment of veterans with disabilities were passed by nations such as Germany in 1919 and 1920, Italy in 1921, and France in 1923 (Kulkarni, 1983:10). Subsequently, in the aftermath of World War II, many countries revised their laws and expanded them to include large numbers of disabled civilians. Other nations including Great Britain joined the list of states which required private employers to hire disabled persons. As a result, a series of laws to promote the employment of disabled citizens were approved in Europe which appeared to be more extensive than comparable measures in the United States.

Public policy concerning disabled persons in most countries is scattered throughout a confusing array of measures and regulations in a manner that seems to resemble the fragmented approach to the study of disability in colleges and universities. Perhaps the most prominent difference between European and American views on the employment of citizens with disabilities, however, is the presence in many European countries of a quota system or laws requiring employers to hire a specified percentage of disabled workers. These provisions contain implications which extend beyond the simple assertion that disabled and nondisabled applicants for a job must be treated equally or even plans which ask employers to take positive steps to increase the number of disabled employees in the work force. While the mandatory nature of quotas obviously may reduce managerial discretion in the selection of personnel, they assume that the hiring of disabled persons is an obligation which can be legitimately imposed on employers and enforced through appropriate penalties. In assigning major responsibility for the employment of disabled citizens to the private labor market, quotas embody a compulsory feature which cannot be found in other policies designed to fulfill similar objectives. Although a partial explanation of the widespread acceptance of quotas undoubtedly can be ascribed to the devastating consequences of the wars which were fought on European soil, this pattern also seems to reflect a natural extension of prevailing concepts of equality and social welfare. The purpose of quotas is not limited to expanding the employment opportunities available to individuals with disabilities; they also might have beneficial effects for a group of people who may be prevented by other aspects of the environment from competing with the nondisabled on an equal basis. As a result, the quota system can be perceived as compensatory effort to balance the relative advantages and disadvantages of disabled and nondisabled segments of society.

American assessments of quotas for the employment of disabled persons in Europe reveal a mixed response. Stubbins (1982) has noted that they are supported by several interest groups in Great Britain. Vash (1980-83), however, seemed to reflect the consensus of opinion accurately when she observed that the quota system simply has not produced the results which it was intended to accomplish. Another perspective has been offered by Kulkarni (1983:67) who concluded, "A balanced policy that aims at providing a supply of well-trained handicapped workers and creates job demand through a legislated quota can provide an ideal solution of the employment problems of disabled persons." In part perhaps American judgments about European quotas have been shaped by the traditional emphasis in the former country on an economic perspective yielding programs of vocational rehabilitation which are designed to offer a large number of well prepared and highly motivated disabled workers to the private labor market. Many Europeans, however, also share the view that the quota system has not worked effectively. A pervasive lack of compliance with existing requirements for hiring persons with disabilities in almost all areas of the world has prevented public policies from exerting any appreciate impact on the rate of unemployment among this portion of the population. But problems of implementation need not be confused with evaluations of the strength or weakness of principles. In fact, employer reluctance to observe regulations concerning the employment of persons with disabilities seems to indicate a need to focus increased attention on administrative issues which might affect the conduct of government programs rather than on the characteristics of disabled individuals or the allegedly inexorable laws which may influence the operation of the economy. Additional efforts, therefore, must be undertaken to assess the potential value of employment quotas as a means of promoting increased equality for citizens with disabilities.

Although European policies were not designed amid a general recognition of persistent patterns of prejudice against disabled citizens, they seem to contain a useful vehicle of promoting the advancement of equal rights for this minority group. Unlike alternative programs which focus almost exclusively on efforts to improve the functional or vocational capabilities of the individual, the quota system appears to offer a valuable method of altering the attitudinal and the man-made environment in which disabled people must seek work. As one of the strongest pieces in the arsenal of weapons which can be used to attack bias and discrimination, quotas can be used as a means of providing increased benefits for disabled workers and of elevating the social and economic status of this segment of the population. Perhaps one of the most remarkable features of European quotas, therefore, is the absence of any significant complaints about reverse discrimination. No major objections have been raised that quotas give disabled persons an unfair advantage in the labor market. This lack of opposition seems especially remarkable in a period of relatively high unemployment. While some observers might argue that this silence is a reflection of the general failure of public officials to enforce the law, this interpretation does not explain the fact that there has been no public disapproval of the quota system in principle. Employment quotas for workers with disabilities do not seem incompatible with the concept of equality. As a result, there appear to be important reasons for conducting a detailed investigation focusing on the application of quotas to the employment problems which confront disabled citizens.

The Study of Employment Policy for Disabled Persons in Europe

An important purpose of this study is to examine European perceptions of employment policy for persons with disabilities. In this research, major attention is devoted to Great Britain, France, West Germany, and Sweden. Of these countries, only Sweden has not adopted a quota system to promote the employment of disabled workers. The primary method used in this investigation was the conduct of interviews with knowledgeable informants about employment policy for disabled citizens. Principal emphasis was placed on the collection of qualitative rather than quantitative data. Although the absence of any means of drawing a random sample of survey respondents precluded the use of statistical measures in the analysis, the information derived from this field work contained a rich lode of insights, observations, and appraisals about the most feasible means of increasing employment of disabled persons.

In each country, appointments were obtained with representatives of four major groups concerned with the employment problems faced by disabled citizens including organizations of disabled persons, voluntary associations or charities, rehabilitation agencies, and government bureaus. Unfortunately, the inclusion of two other important groups concerned with the hiring of disabled people, trade unions and employers, was precluded by the limitations of time and resources. More than thirty in-depth interviews were conducted with persons involved in this issue to secure their perceptions of the strengths and weaknesses of employment policies for persons with disabilities in each of the four countries. Since prior discussions of this issue have tended to revolve around the opinions of rehabilitation professionals, government officials, and spokespersons for voluntary organizations, major attention in this study is devoted to the views and assessments of the leaders of organizations of people with disabilities.

One of the most significant findings of the research was the degree of unanimity which existed among representatives of each of the four major groups included in the study. Most of the leaders of organizations of disabled persons tended to endorse some type of quota system to promote the employment of disabled workers. Less support for this position was found among the representatives of rehabilitation agencies, government administrators, and voluntary associations. This result seemed to reinforce the distinction between organizations ''of and for'' people with disabilities which was made repeatedly by disabled Europeans. Despite the appearance that disabled people sometimes lack unity and cohesion, the amount of agreement produced by this issue seemed to indicate the presence of a disability perspective, or a distinctive set of values related to extensive experience with a disability, which may eventually become an important political force in many nations of the world.

Disabled persons generally favored a compulsory approach to employment which differed significantly from the voluntary, discretionary, or programmatic nature of most of the alternatives proposed by rehabilitation agencies, public officials, or organizations dominated by nondisabled members. This pattern appears to lend support to the interpretation that disabled people increasingly perceive the solution to employment problems as part of a broader struggle to gain equal rights rather than as a form of help or assistance which can be provided by public or private institutions.

Perhaps most importantly, the convergence of opinions among the leaders of organizations of disabled persons in various countries exceeded the harmony displayed by disabled leaders, rehabilitation professionals, government personnel, and representatives of voluntary associations within each nation. While the residents of separate countries naturally might be expected to express favorable viewpoints about policies adopted by their homeland, the results of this investigation appear to suggest that the affinities inspired by the role of a disability advocate or activist may be an even more crucial determinant of a disabled person's sentiments about salient political issues than the allegiances produced by citizenship. Even in Sweden, which has displayed exceptional pride in the programs that it has established for the disability community, representatives of organizations of disabled citizens and other individuals with disabilities confided that the continuing problem of unemployment might eventually lead them to support mandatory programs for the hiring of disabled workers such as a quota system. As a result, primary emphasis in this research also is placed on the distinction between the perceptions of leaders of organizations of disabled persons and other observers rather than on the differences between the four nations.

Nonetheless, laws and regulations concerning disabled citizens in every country of Europe obviously have reflected important variations in cultural values and traditions. Since policies affecting the employment of disabled persons generally were not developed until the twentieth century, for example, national legacies established by charitable organizations in the nineteenth century or earlier have seemed to produce differences in the definition of public and private responsibilities for meeting the needs of citizens with disabilities (Kramer, 1981). In order to encapsulate some of the most crucial dimensions of employment policies for disabled workers in Great Britain, France, West Germany, and Sweden, therefore, a brief summary of major characteristics of laws and policies regarding this issue has been prepared for each nation.

The British approach seemingly can be characterized as a form of welfare pluralism or differentiated support which is associated with (a) relatively ambiguous operational definitions of disability; (b) a quota system perceived by many observers as unattainable and unenforceable; (c) a registration process widely viewed as necessary but based on few incentives; (d) the imposition of relatively few rewards or penalties in the implementation of employment policies; (e) education and training programs comparable with those established in other advanced industrialized nations; (f) the initiation of efforts to improve accessibility and transportation facilities; (g) a network of sheltered workshops proportionate to perceived needs; and (h) a high rate of unemployment among disabled persons.

The French perspective seems to reflect a form of protective assistance which is related to (a) relatively wide discretion in the definition of disability; (b) a quota commonly regarded as too high; (c) ambivalence about registration; (d) penalties sometimes viewed as too severe; (e) relatively extensive support for education and training programs; (f) a somewhat vague promise of increased accessibility and transportation for disabled citizens; (g) a prominent role for sheltered workshops; and (h) comparatively high rates of unemployment in the disability community.

The German emphasis on a bureaucratic approach of technical rationality appears to embody (a) strict medical and economic definitions of disability; (b) major reliance on a quota system to increase the employment of disabled persons; (c) a system of registration, which is still sharply questioned, based on numerous incentives; (d) a penalty widely regarded as too low; (e) a major stress on education and training programs; (f) a moderate focus on accessibility and transportation issues; (g) reducing the role of sheltered workshops; and (h) a relatively high level of unemployment among disabled persons.

The Swedish model of subsidization in a professionalized community seems to encompass (a) pragmatic and expansive definitions of disability; (b) the use of economic incentives rather than coercion to promote the employment of disabled workers; (c) a registration system implying many benefits and relatively little stigma; (d) offers of positive enticements for hiring disabled personnel; (e) plans to make sheltered workshops increasingly competitive; (f) widespread education and training programs; (g) comparatively advanced accessibility and transportation policies; and (h) levels of unemployment among disabled citizens which is perceived as unduly high.

Although national traditions obviously have produced some variations in employment policies for disabled citizens, these patterns do not seem to reflect important differences in prevalent European understandings of the concept of equality. In each of the countries, governments have played a major role in efforts to improve the social and economic position of people with disabilities. In order to assess the combination of policy characteristics which is most likely to promote increased equality for disabled persons, therefore, all of the major components of the issue will be examined individually rather than within the context of separate nations.

SECTION FOUR: PERCEPTIONS OF EUROPEAN EMPLOYMENT FOR THE DISABLED

In the formulation of public policy, conflict and discord about alternative methods of achieving desired goals tend to be the rule rather than the exception. People who are most directly affected by political decisions have separate interests which naturally yield different perceptions about the details of government programs. Although knowledgeable observers in Europe were strongly committed to the increased employment of disabled persons, for example, there were important disagreements about the most effective means of achieving that objective. In this discussion, initial attention is directed at general assessments of the strengths and weaknesses of employment policies for people with disabilities and subsequent consideration is given to specific controversies raised by this issue.

In European nations, the employment of disabled workers commonly is viewed as part of a broader duty of government and the society. In France, observers often spoke of the responsibilities of the "collectivity." In Sweden, comparable emphasis was placed on the concept of "solidarity." As a government officer in France explained, "The principle is that, being handicapped, you have a right from the collectivity to be helped...Children will be educated and adults who don't work will be granted an allowance based on their own position, not the position of the family." A prominent public official in Sweden pointed out that disability programs in that country emerged from the political parties, unions, and organizations of disabled people which "found a common or...solidary policy in which employers have to pay attention to...social factors and societal responsibility and take factors other than merit into account." As a nondisabled spokesperson for a large organization of disabled persons in Sweden said, "The idea is that handicapped people should live as normally as possible." The principle of societal responsibility implied of such statements, therefore, seems to reflect a sharp contrast to American concerns about the notion of individualism.

Yet these approaches have not necessarily attracted strong approval from the disability community. A French leader of an organization of disabled citizens noted, "There is a philosophical problem. In France, a large part of the parents and social workers think a handicapped person cannot work in an ordinary situation so the effort of the collectivity is placed on 'special workers.' ...The consequence is that handicapped persons are denied access to professional education." As a rehabilitation worker acknowledged, " The French mentality considers different or disabled people as persons they must assist." Similarly, a disability activist in Sweden observed, "The Social Democratic party since the nineteen-thirties had a lot of redistributive programs so they could not overlook the disabled. In fact, they've used us as an appeal for solidarity, which is just another name for charity... In Sweden, they give disabled people things only as part of a general plan." Thus, many of these criticisms seem to reflect a belief that, in the desire to aid disabled citizens, governments and societies often impose limitations on personal capacities which are not necessarily implied by their disabilities. As the same Swedish activist stated, "I wouldn't call it paternalism, which to me sounds too personal for what is going on here. Here it's a question of professionalism. They consider you an object of their professional activities. The issue is your choice versus their planning, bureaucratic procedures, and professional attitudes."

Perhaps part of the objections to government policy voiced by persons with disabilities reflected a basic dissatisfaction with administrative practices. As a disabled leader in West Germany stated, "In Germany, disability is a technical issue...So if people have an education, everything is well organized by the government. And then you're on your own living in a society that tries to solve problems in technical ways rather than in terms of attitudes." Another disabled leader in Germany pointed out that government programs typically assume that "they know what's good for disabled people."

A similar theme was expressed by several leaders of organizations of disabled persons in Great Britain. As one said, "We accept the welfare state as a basis for a humane approach, but it tends to be paternalistic and bureaucratic. We are concerned with the question: How can the welfare tradition become more responsive to disabled people? We want to reorganize the welfare state to make clients a part of the fabric." Another disabled leader in that country expressed the hope that organizations of people with disabilities might eventually develop an interlocking network with a possible veto power in the social service infrastructure. Although much of the energy of organizations of disabled persons in Great Britain recently has concentrated on efforts to retain the quota system and to introduce anti-discrimination legislature, the eventual goals of many disabled persons seem to extend far beyond these objectives. As an additional disabled leader proposed, "The short-run problem is how to get as much as you can from the system, and the long-term solution is to change the economic system. In the short-term, you sometimes have to work in counter-productive directions. Anti-discrimination legislation is a prime example. This legislation can only be granted as an accommodation to existing social relations. There is a need for broader changes in the ways in which disabled people relate to the productive process...We cannot long afford to be a special category that people can make allowances for." Many leaders of the social and political movement of disabled persons in France, Sweden, West Germany, and Great Britain seemed to share a conviction that there is a need for sweeping changes not only in government programs but also in the values and structures of society.

There is often an important relationship between general perspectives on social issues and operational definitions of the problem. In the case of employment policies for disabled persons, many programs have apparently floundered on the lack of a clear and unambiguous definition of disability. Perhaps the most meaningful distinction between the criteria used in European countries can be expressed as the difference between the German approach, which is based on somewhat technical medical and economic considerations, and the more nebulous guidelines adopted by Sweden, France, and Great Britain.

In West Germany, disability generally is determined by a list of functional impairments which is related to economic considerations. A distinction is made between disabled and severely disabled individuals based upon a fifty percent capacity to work. As one leader of an organization of disabled Germans put it, "Basically, the medical model is the same as you have it in the United States. The most widely used legal definition is 'the reduction of the capability to earn an income,' which is the basis for compensation and benefits." Although acknowledging difficulties with the standard, the same spokesperson was reluctant to change it. As he said, "At some point, they want to substitute 'degree of disability' for 'diminished earning capacity.' …I fear they will take away some rights because they will say that, when you are able to work, you do not need any financial help. The disabled organizations say only that we need a new word for disability in a social context; and some people misunderstand this…We say that you need a balance for your disadvantages…One problem is that we speak about social rehabilitation, but we do not have it." Although this leader felt that medical and economic definitions could be used as a foundation for combating the social problems confronted by people with disabilities, he also appeared to welcome a new definition which might gain general acceptance. Like advocates for many organizations of disabled persons in Europe, however, he appeared to express the feeling that he was frequently placed on the defensive in his negotiations with other influential groups in the political process.

Perhaps the broadest and most expansive definition of disability can be found in Sweden. As one government administrator expressed it, "A person is handicapped in the labor market if he has problems getting or keeping a job. It depends on the regional economy, training, and many other things." Social disabilities such as alcoholism or drug abuse also are included in the determinations made by the labor market board. Another public official concluded, "The main answer is that we have a pragmatic way of doing it… There is no line separating the disabled and the nondisabled." Some persons praised this approach. As a spokesperson for sheltered workshops said, "Sweden does not have a concept of productive capacity. That is a way of classifying people. I don't like it. They are labeled quite enough." Others, however, displayed reservations. As a Swedish representative of an organization of disabled people put it, "The politicians do good things, but they are widening the definition so that resources don't come down to us. I would very much relate that problem to the definition."

There is also vast discretion in the definitions of disability used in France. A French government official noted, "The 1975 act created in each department or county a commission for handicapped adults where they can apply for help. The commission decides the degree of handicap and if you can work...If the person can and wants to work, he may be sent to an education or training center, a sheltered workshop, or ordinary employment.'' This approach was criticized by a rehabilitation agency which sought to replace it with an essentially economic definition. ''For us, a handicap is an aptitude just below the norm and not a type of impairment. Our perspective is a management rather than a medical or diagnostic approach which is not operation in the firm and introduces notions which are not necessary.'' Perhaps even more telling were the objections of a French leader of an organization of disabled persons who commented, ''In France, the local commissions decide who is disabled, and they determine productive capacity; but the members know nothing about the problems of disability because they have never worked where disabled people are employed.''

The exercise of discretion and the effort to include labor market considerations in administrative standards also have created definitional difficulties in Great Britain. One disabled spokesperson for a voluntary organization pointed out that the problem of developing a definition matters a great deal because of proposals to provide a disability allowance to compensate disabled citizens for the extra costs which they must incur due to their disabilities. As he observed, ''There is no definition of disability so the government can't calculate the costs, and they won't introduce the program...The local authorities have a very open-ended policy such that anyone who is so disabled that he needs benefits must be disabled. They drive a wedge between us in order to manipulate us.'' A representative of a British rehabilitation agency also concluded, ''The definition is at fault at the end of the day. The Manpower Services Commission does not issue guidelines to Disablement Resettlement Offices because they say the definition should depend upon changes in the job market.''

Despite these problems, there appeared to be strong support for mandatory employment quotas among organizations of disabled persons and other groups in many European countries. In Great Britain, for example, these organizations have been involved in a successful effort to defeat a recent proposal by the Manpower Services Commission (1979) to eliminate the quota system. As one spokesperson for an organization of disabled persons stated, ''The government said the quota doesn't work, but we are now reviewing it because the minister says it is going to stay...We caused a fuss, the disabled got together, and the government realized that there was not the support for eliminating it that the government claimed.'' While some British voluntary organizations preferred an emphasis on job placement efforts or increased economic incentives for employers to promote the hiring of disabled workers, most organizations of people with disabilities in Great Britain and elsewhere appeared to be united in their support of some type of quota system to secure increased equality for this segment of the population.

A major part of the controversy over the quota system seems to revolve about administrative issues. Massie (1982) has noted that bulk permits exempting corporations from the requirement to hire disabled workers have been showered on British employers like "confetti at a...wedding." The Manpower Services Commission has estimated that a ten percent reduction in the issuance of bulk permits might require a major increase in staff and expenditures. But this action also could produce a significant expansion of job opportunities for disabled persons.

In addition, Noble (1982) has warned that the use of a quota system or similar measures could prompt an effort by employers to redefine the physical characteristics of their workers in order to meet the requirements imposed by law. Yet extensive questioning about this issue among rehabilitation agencies, voluntary organizations, government officials, and organizations of people with disabilities in many areas of Europe failed to disclose any detectable evidence of this practice. With the exception of some disabled leaders who noted that job applicants with slight disabilities often are preferred, there appeared too few indications that employers had engaged in a systematic attempt to circumvent quotas in this manner.

Moreover, similar investigations failed to reveal any reports of resentment among nondisabled employees concerning the preferential treatment granted to disabled persons under the quota system. Despite the definitional ambiguities produced by a lack of clear standards for determining disability, employment quotas for disabled workers have not appeared to create many problems which might otherwise have been predicted. Perhaps this pattern has resulted from a general failure to enforce the provisions of the quota system, or perhaps a disability is commonly perceived as so stigmatizing that few are prepared to question the benefits granted to disabled citizens. Conceivably, these facts may be associated with other interpretations which have not yet been identified. As a French leader of an organization of disabled persons estimated, "It's in the imagination. Five percent of the employees in an enterprise have an attitude of welcome, five percent treat disabled people like a racist, and ninety percent are unable to form an attitude because, for so many generations, they learned that the problems of the disabled are complex and medicalized. And so they thought disability was a professional problem and not their own problem." In any event, the findings suggest that there do not seem to be insurmountable barriers to the adoption of quotas to promote the employment of citizens with disabilities.

Perhaps a major difficulty impeding the effectiveness of quotas concerns the administrative organization of agencies responsible for its implementation. In Great Britain, for example, this duty is vested in the Manpower Services Commission, which has sought to divest itself of the task by urging the repeal of he quota system, and in its employees, the Disablement Resettlement Officers, who have direct contact with disabled citizens and representatives of employers. These officers are required to enforce the quotas and to engage in job placement efforts on behalf of their clients. Since persons responsible for hiring workers seem to offer the most immediate prospects for fulfilling their obligations, some have suggested that the DROs identify more closely with employers than with disabled persons. This tendency may be endemic to any programs based on job placement activities. As one British leader of an organization of disabled citizens put it, ''They don't like being policemen and advocates. They feel embarrassed with personnel officers.'' As long as increasing the employment of people with disabilities are viewed primarily as an attempt to persuade employers to hire another disabled worker rather than as an effort to secure equal rights for members of this minority, the enforcement of legal requirements may remain a secondary goal for personnel involved in this issue.

There are, however, other important questions which must be considered in the administration of employment policies for disabled persons. One such dimension is the problem of registration. In Great Britain, lack of compliance with the quota system often has been related to the reluctance of many persons to register as disabled workers. While some have interpreted this reticence as reflecting a desire to avoid the stigma of a disability, many British activists point out that present policies provide few incentives to register as a disabled person. As one member of the Association of Disabled Professionals stated at a meeting, ''Because you can't get jobs, no one registers. If registration did produce jobs, people would be crawling out from the rocks to register.'' Another disabled spokesperson for a voluntary organization noted that registration rates are much higher among persons with visual impairments who are provided with a broader range of services than people with other types of disabilities.

Similarly, in Germany, where national guilt about the extermination of one million disabled citizens during the Nazi regime has raised dire fears about registration and about the general discussion of other disability issues, important incentives apparently have been sufficient to overcome the anxieties of disabled persons. As a disabled leader noted, ''The fears seem to be among the officials and not among the handicapped.'' Even a government administrator acknowledged, ''If you want to be registered, you must go and ask for it. If you do that, you can go by bus without paying and you can take six more days of holiday. So nearly everyone asks for such a paper.''

In Sweden, which does not have a quota system, disabled individuals may register at employment offices to obtain assistance in securing jobs. Yet, even here, bureaucrats may feel the desire to maintain good relations with employers who might be able to help them with future placement efforts. As one spokesperson for a Swedish organization of disabled persons observed, ''There is a lack of courage. They can't decide whose side they're on.'' The potential pro-employer bias of persons engaged in job placement, therefore, appears to be a greater source of concern in Europe than in the United States.

Probably the most unusual form of quotas can be found in France which has a system of "reserved employment" requiring employers who do not fulfill the quota to reserve a future job opening for a disabled worker. When the designated position becomes vacant, employers are required to consult the local commission for adults with disabilities to determine whether or not a disabled person is available to fill the slot. This approach has drawn sharp criticism from a rehabilitation agency which stated, "It is important to transform the reserved position to [a requirement stipulating] the number of disabled people who must be employed. We would prefer to have a number rather than a specific post designated…It is a handicap for disabled people because the firms are obliged to restrict disabled persons to a specific post… There is no harmony between the disabled people who they are searching for and the administration's ability to find good people or to put the right people in the right place…Every post can be occupied by a disabled person. It's ridiculous." Nonetheless, the spokesperson for this agency went on to underscore its support for the principle of quotas, "We think it's important to have a law to oblige firms because in France we are not ready to act without obligation. We are critics of the process but not of the obligation." Similar sentiments were expressed by the leader of a French organization of disabled citizens who stated, "We think we must preserve the quota because it is the only way to remind business enterprises and public opinion that many disabled people want to work."

Another important issue in the development of a quota system is the determination of the percentage of disabled workers which an employer can be required to hire. Quotas can be used as a target to stimulate increased employment or an irreducible minimum below which this proportion cannot fall. Since there is a lack of compliance with quota provisions in many European countries, this question has not received extensive attention. In France, however, an official of a rehabilitation agency complained that the quota percentage, which seemed to be based on the number of persons disabled in war plus the number of civilians with disabilities, has "no sociological context…There are not enough disabled people to fill the quota." In West Germany, a government official also commented, "We have to think about a higher percentage. The trade unions are trying to get a higher levy. But this government does not want it, because they say we have to do more for the employer to get a better economy. We are thinking of increasing both the levy and the percentage, but I think we can sooner raise the percentage." Like most other political issues, decisions about the size of the quota for employing disabled workers may be determined by the relative strength of powerful interest groups. As this official also admitted, "Right now, the employers are stronger on this issue." Whether or not the proposed change will have the intended effect of increasing employment for disabled citizens, however, remains problematic.

Perhaps the most critical features of the quota system are the penalties or rewards which can be imposed to enforce its provisions. In Great Britain, employers who fail to meet the quota are subject to criminal proceedings; but only nine prosecutions have been brought against six firms since 1947 (Kulkarni, 1983:27). In France, failure to fulfill quota obligations can result in heavy fines; but many observers complain that these penalties are too high. In West Germany, compliance with the quota is enforced by a social levy, or an equalization payment used partially to finance the rehabilitation of other disabled persons, which many regard as too low. And in Sweden, which does not have a quota system, numerous spokespersons criticized the lack of effective instruments to require the employment of disabled workers. The problem of developing appropriate administrative mechanisms to insure that employers respect their legal responsibilities, therefore, is central to evaluations of the quota system.

The relative ineffectiveness of criminal prosecution in the British experience has prompted a search for other means of securing observance of the law. As one British leader of an organization of disabled persons stated, ''The government has been trying to abolish the quota scheme. Some say it is sabotage. There is no intention of prosecuting. But there has got to be a firm legislative basis requiring employers to hire disabled workers. I believe the quota can have some effect, but I'm also in favor of antidiscrimination legislation.'' Another disabled spokesperson for a voluntary association said, ''Right now we could do with a bit of positive discrimination. Three years ago, I wouldn't have said that.''

These views were not necessarily shared by some nondisabled representatives of voluntary groups in Great Britain. One such observer commented, ''The government sees quotas as restraints on employers and constraints on the free market. There will be no change in enforcement because there is no commitment to it at the highest levels…I don't think the Manpower Services Commission can stand accused, even by the most strident organizations, of breaking its own rules. In theory, you could devise water-tight rules; but then you run into problems of political expediency especially in the current economic climate. The future lies in multiplying effective incentives for employers rather than multiplying coercion.'' Another nondisabled employee of a voluntary association commented, ''I favor the quota scheme to the levy scheme because many people would pay the fine rather than following the law. The levy scheme seems to be saying that disabled people are not such good employees. The quota doesn't imply that.'' Yet perhaps the predominate consensus of opinion on this issue was expressed by a spokesperson for a British rehabilitation agency in saying, ''Personally, I favor a levy system. There should be strict penalties with enforcement by an impartial independent body…There is also a good case to be made for antidiscrimination legislation. I would like to see it included in the context of a quota system.''

Although the legal climate of Sweden has not been conducive to development of a quota system or antidiscrimination statutes, many commentators in that country have raised serious questions about the effectiveness of existing measures to secure the employment of disabled persons. A government administrator described the Swedish approach by saying, "If an employer does not have a socially responsible attitude toward hiring handicapped people, we can take up discussions with the employer...It's an alternative to the quota system." Another public official reported that, even though Sweden opted to provide economic stimulation for employers and extensive resources for disabled individuals rather than employment quotas, "We have a powerful system of whips and carrots, but we still have problems." The same theme was echoed by an employee of an organization of disabled persons: "We have the carrot, but we need more pressure." But a disabled spokesperson for another organization of citizens with disabilities eventually concluded, "I don't have the answer on how the forcing system should be carried out—by setting up a...percentage requirement or by stimulating employers financially. We have tried the cooperative method and failed. I think in a few years we will be demanding the quota system perhaps combined with some financial stimulation to the employer."

In France, by contrast, existing provisions for the enforcement of the quota system is widely perceived as too severe. As a government official admitted, "If you don't respect the quota, there might be a heavy penalty. That's the reason it's not enforced. It's too heavy." Some French rehabilitation agencies reported that they had also attempted unsuccessfully to introduce a levy system based on the German model. Others remarked that many employers continued to pay the fines and to exclude disabled persons from the labor force because of a reluctance to modify the worksite, trade union opposition, and other reasons. As the leader of a French organization of disabled persons commented, "If an industry cannot find a disabled worker and doesn't try, they must pay a high penalty...But often industry prefers to pay the tax rather than to employ disabled people."

While the levy system of enforcing employment quotas in West Germany was widely supported by organizations of disabled citizens and other observers throughout Europe, many persons also noted that the penalty of that country was not high enough to produce the desired result. An estimated one-third of the German firms covered by this law do not employ a single worker with a severe disability (Kulkarni, 1983:22). The amount of the levy, which is 100 marks or approximately 55 dollars per month for each position in the quota that remains unfilled, is often regarded by German employers as a charitable contribution or as a normal business expense. As a leader of a German organization of disabled persons commented, "When employers pay 100 marks, it is really 50 marks because they don't pay taxes on the position. So, therefore, it is cheap for the employer to pay the levy and not hire disabled people." As a result, some organizations, including German trade unions, have proposed that the levy should be raised automatically in relation to changing economic conditions.

The size of a penalty imposed for failure to comply with a legal requirement must be considered as independent of the principle upon which the law is based. Presumably, if an economy is assumed to be competitive, there should be some level at which the costs of a penalty imposed for failure to hire disabled workers might affect the price of goods and thereby the competitive position of a business in the marketplace. Perhaps one of the major responsibilities of policy-makers, professionals, and consumers is to seek to identify the level at which the costs of excluding disabled workers exceed the advantages of ignoring legal responsibilities in the context of a policy which views the employment of disabled persons as a legitimate obligation rather than as a charitable act or an unrealistic expectation. Although cost-benefit calculations do not encompass other important legislative intentions such as efforts to combat discrimination or attempts to achieve increased equality, these techniques seemingly could be used as a method of devising appropriate remedies for an apparent reticence to fulfill mandated objectives. The problems of implementing a quota system do not appear to be insurmountable. Instead, these difficulties seem to revolve about administrative issues which may reflect the intensity of a commitment to the goal of promoting increased employment for citizens with disabilities.

Perhaps the principal alternatives to mandatory plans such as the quota system are government subsidies for employers who agree to facilitate the hiring of disabled workers. Each of the four European countries has experimented with some form of this approach. Yet there does not appear to be definitive empirical evidence or unanimity in the assessment of the policy. Like many other political issues, opinions about compulsory employment quotas or economic incentives for hiring disabled persons seem to reflect basic disagreements about social and economic values. While subsidies for employers attracted the most support from government officials and voluntary associations, many organizations of people with disabilities and others expressed objections to these programs.

The basic issue involved in policies to provide economic incentives for the employment of disabled persons was reflected in a question posed by a government administrator in Sweden: "If an employer has a choice between a young worker and a handicapped worker with a seventy-five percent subsidy, which will he choose?" Although the answer may not be obvious, many countries have endorsed financial support to offset alleged differences between the productive capacities of disabled and nondisabled workers. As another public official in Sweden suggested, "We know that all people are not equal in productive capacity, and the payment is based on this expectation." Even in France, the government is experimenting with on-the-job training and other programs to compensate for the supposed deficiencies of disabled workers. Arguments for employment subsidies also are based on concepts of efficiency. As a spokesperson for voluntary organizations in Great Britain stated, "Perhaps the only realistic and moral way to define employment rights is to determine available resources, work democratically, and develop priorities.'' From this perspective, the preference for employer subsidies may reflect an assumption that they are more likely to contribute to economic growth and development than enforcement of the quota system.

In response, the leaders of organizations of disabled persons and others often question assumptions about the association between disability and work capacities upon which much social welfare legislation appears to be founded. One British leader commented, ''The government has adopted a job introduction scheme for six weeks. There are very few figures on how successful it is. According to Mrs. Thatcher, we should give more money to disabled people who can't work. But we're really going back to Victorian values. There is a chapter in [a recent government report on education for disabled students] on 'significant living without work.' But disabled people… don't want 'significant living without work' while everyone else is working.'' Another rehabilitation professional in Great Britain observed, ''I don't like the concept of subsidizing employment because it conveys the idea that employers are doing something special.'' In West Germany, a leader of an organization of disabled citizens noted that subsidized employment based on a trial period of work, ''Often creates problems because it is not easy to live when you do not know if you can keep the post or not.'' Even a government official in Germany admitted that the success of subsidized employment depends mainly on ''the promise of the employer.'' Moreover a spokesperson for a Swedish organization of disabled persons reported that increases in economic incentives for employers have not produced significant gains in the employment of disabled persons: ''We have increased the subsidies, but the results are worse.''

Many objections to the enforcement of quotas for hiring disabled persons appeared to reflect assumptions about the scarcity of resources during a period of fiscal stringency and relatively high unemployment. Yet there are no assurances that alternatives—and seemingly less expensive—programs will produce substantial benefits for citizens with disabilities. As one leader of an organization of disabled persons in Sweden put it, ''The government has attempted to increase the employment of disabled workers by appealing to the national conscience, but unemployed youth are more dangerous to them.'' Without an extensive reexamination of the employment problems facing citizens with disabilities or a significant change in the social and political influence available to them, there is a serious threat that programs based solely on an altruistic desire to assist disabled workers might fail to fulfill the needs of this segment of the population. In the allocation of funds for employment subsidies and similar policies, persons with disabilities often are placed at a serious disadvantage.

The choice between employment subsidies and quotas appears to be founded, in large measure, on competing economic and legal theories. While the proponents of subsidies for employers generally believe that economic stimulation is the best method of reducing unemployment among disabled persons and other groups, advocates who stress measures such as the quota system often present arguments that reflect a broader range of considerations. In part, this controversy represents political disagreements. As a rehabilitation professional in West Germany observed, "The conservative government feels that forcing employment is not the right way and favors education and voluntary action. Their opponents support increased levies." In addition, however, proposals for economic incentives seem to suggest that encouraging or inducing employers to hire disabled workers is the most effective method of achieving this policy objective. By contrast, quotas imply a duty or an obligation to fulfill the goal. These contrasts appear to reflect fundamental differences not only about the extent to which disability is defined by functional impairments and vocational limitations or by bias and discrimination but also about individualistic and collective approaches to the solution of social problems. While employment subsidies may be interpreted primarily as an effort to offset the personal restrictions of a disability, quotas seem to be more compatible with a perspective that regards discrimination as the major problem confronting disabled persons. In a political system committed to providing equal rights for all citizens, an exclusive reliance on economic blandishments might not be considered an appropriate way of combatting prejudice and segregation. Similarly, whereas incentives or persuasion focus principally on attempts to change the practices of individual employers, quotas seem to rest upon a belief that extensive governmental intervention may be required to secure increased employment for citizens with disabilities. Means usually are inextricably related to ends. Decisions about alternative approaches to employment policies for disabled persons, therefore, cannot be divorced from a broader examination of social and political values.

Although controversies about subsidies and quotas appeared to represent a major source of conflict about efforts to increase employment for disabled persons, these approaches do not encompass all of the programs which had been adopted by European countries to fulfill this goal. The prospects of securing employment available to disabled citizens in different nations also are affected by policies concerning sheltered workshops, education or training, transportation, attendants, accessibility, and other issues. In many of these areas, European commitments to the objective of providing equal treatment for people with disabilities seem to exceed advances made in the United States. A prominent public official in Sweden, for example, described that country's approach to the problem of securing an accessible environment by saying, "There are two principles of responsibility and finance which I call 'the natural way.' The first states that anyone responsible for providing a service must be certain that it is accessible to disabled people. The other principle of finance says that the cost of making it available to disabled persons should be considered the natural cost of the product. We try to see that these principles are carried through." While the principal immediate effects of this policy are imposed upon consumers who purchase goods in the private sector, their long-term influence on employment opportunities for disabled persons in an increasingly barrier-free environment may be extensive. Despite important variations in national programs affecting such issues, however, they have not yet appeared to produce a significant impact on the programs encountered by disabled persons in seeking jobs.

One important element of European policies which may deserve more intensive study in the United States, however, is the widespread provision of governmental support to compensate disabled citizens for the additional costs produced by a disability. In addition to medical care, disabled persons in several countries are granted a mobility allowance and other assistance to help defray the extra expenses which they must assume in order to become independent participants in the life of the society. As one leader of a German organization of disabled citizens commented, ''Disabled people have to spend more than the nondisabled. In Germany, the government makes an effort to make up the difference in costs.'' Much of the debate about these policies has focused on the question of whether or not they should be subject to a ''means test,'' or criteria based on the ability of a disabled individual to pay for these expenses. As another German leader stated, ''The general rule is that attendant care and other services may be subsidized if you are very rich or very poor. For the broad group of middle-income people, it's a problem.'' Perhaps the most extensive proposals on this issue have been introduced in Great Britain where some groups have suggested that the government should provide a general disability allowance as compensation for the added costs incurred by disabled persons. As one British leader of an organization of disabled citizens stated, ''We're coming close to all parties agreeing to some kind of disability allowance which would be equivalent to the benefits provided industrially injured workers, but it won't happen soon...There would be no means test, and recipients would be allowed to work. People have to accept a lot of additional expenses because of a disability...Studies of this are beginning; but some have found that, because many disabled persons have such little money, they are not able to afford many extra costs. On the other hand, the more income disabled people have, the more they spend on aspects of their lives affected by the disability.'' The provision of various types of disability allowances obviously represents an important step toward increased equality for disabled persons. Yet, while this type of support offers further incentives for people with disabilities to pursue jobs and to earn higher incomes, it does not remove the discriminatory barriers which have often frustrated their efforts to gain employment. Disability may reflect an employment problem which cannot be solved without a significant expansion of legal rights as well as economic benefits.

In spite of the numerous policies which have been approved to promote the employment of disabled people in Europe, the problem appears to be a troubling enigma for many public decision-makers and other interested parties. Available evidence indicates that, in European countries, unemployment rates for disabled persons are extraordinarily high and comparable to estimated levels in the United States. Many of the potential pitfalls of the examination of unemployment figures, which might be considered the appropriate dependent variable for any assessment of employment policies, reflect statistical difficulties produced by different definitions and measures of disability. In France, the estimates of unemployment provided by government officials, rehabilitation agencies, and leaders of organizations of disabled people ranged from two-thirds to three-fourths. In West Germany, most observers acknowledged that the unemployment rate for disabled workers was higher, and perhaps considerably higher, than the equivalent percentage for the nondisabled. In Great Britain, disabled leaders were sharply cirtical of efforts by government agencies to avoid the discussion of unemployment data by focusing on the quality of their job placement activities. And even in Sweden, where a general unemployment rate of three or four percent is widely viewed as too high, a public official, noting that seventy percent of the members of an organization of blind persons were not working in the labor force, candidly admitted, ''We have not been able to produce better employment figures than other countries.'' In fact, none of the informants contacted in this study attempted to claim that the unemployment rate for disabled citizens of any particular country was lower than levels which might be found elsewhere. Nor did anyone deny the seriousness of the problems created by exceptionally high unemployment among this segment of the population. In the context of existing policies, therefore, the employment of disabled persons continues to be an elusive objective.

The image of employment policy for disabled people in Europe appears to reflect a picture of many important laws which remain unenforced and many significant objectives which are still unfulfilled. In these circumstances, therefore, some leaders of organizations of citizens with disabilities have begun to seek alliances with other groups to enhance their political strength and to promote the attainment of their goals. Since employer resistance to compliance with the quota system and other measures has been a major obstacle to the hiring of disabled workers, many leaders of organizations of disabled persons have begun to look to labor unions for support and assistance. As one British leader concluded, ''Quotas would have worked if the trade unions had insisted that they work...The trade union movement has always had a conscience, but it has only started to function in the last fifteen years or so.'' Another British described the position of the unions somewhat more pessimistically by saying ''Their attitude about the quota scheme is somewhat ambivalent. I think the situation will get worse as unemployment worsens. The unions are going to be more concerned about protecting the jobs of their members.''

Skepticism about the role of unions was also expressed in France. As a leader of an organization of disabled persons stated, ''The trade unions and parents have paternalistic ideas which say that handicapped workers in an enterprise will be so exploited that we are marginalized for our own protection." A French spokesperson for a voluntary organization related the criticism of unions to a complaint about quotas by saying, "The main problem is with the unions rather than the employer...Employment rights cannot be touched. The bosses fear that, if they negotiate something for the handicapped, it might become a right...The quota system creates the fear of another right."

Although evidence of increasing cooperation with trade unions was uncovered in West Germany and Sweden, labor did not escape criticism in those countries either. A Swedish leader of an organization of disabled persons noted that government policies have often prevented them from becoming active in labor unions and gaining an improved understanding of their position: "People getting a pension are not getting jobs, so they are not union members. In our contracts with the labor movement, we often meet the attitude: 'isn't it good that they have a pension?'" A public official noted, however, that a strong link is forming between organizations of disabled persons and trade unions because "there is less of a tradition of private charities in Sweden." Similarly, a government official in Germany commented, "The associations of the handicapped and the unions stand together and the employers are opposed. The churches and the charities are indifferent to the matter of the quota system and the levy...They say a lot about education and handicapped workshops. But they don't want the government to do their work." Despite the tension between unions and disabled citizens, many activists seemed to view the labor movement as a more valuable potential ally than many groups which traditionally offered assistance to persons with disabilities.

The social and political movement of citizens with disabilities has not yet emerged as an independent force capable of gaining the recognition and respect of more established interest groups in most European countries. In Great Britain, leaders of organizations of disabled persons complained that they did not represent a powerful constituency. French leaders lamented their inability to change votes between the political left and the right. And, in West Germany, broad organizations of persons with disabilities are still somewhat overshadowed by the relatively limited concerns of larger and more influential groups of disabled veterans. In Sweden, however, which was called a "promised land" of groups where the government subsidizes organizations of disabled citizens, a public official reported that he had been involved in forming "a committee of peoples' movements including unions, renters, disabled persons, and pensioners, which represented 3 million of 8.2 million people in Sweden." But another spokesperson for a Swedish organization of disabled persons pointed out, "Somewhere between ten and twenty percent of handicapped people are members of the handicapped movement. That has very much to do with denying that they are handicapped." The social stigma of disability, which has traditionally impeded the willingness to assume an identification as a disabled person and to mobilize politically to further the interests of this segment of the population, can be a powerful determinant of human behavior. Personal and political battles often are fought at the cost of great psychological anguish. Yet the potential strength of the movement of disabled citizens, based on their own numbers and the size of other groups who share their interests, might eventually become a crucial source of influence in many countries.

The struggle by disabled citizens to gain increased equality has not been without its detractors. As a government employee in Great Britain said, "There are some disabled persons who feel they're owed more than they are given...They are trying to get rid of the British stiff upper lip. They are making disabled people suddenly militant in a rather sour way." These criticisms, however, need not deter citizens with disabilities from the pursuit of significant political goals. In fact, in an atmosphere in which the demands of disabled persons are more often ignored than debated, such opposition might be welcomed as a point of departure for the initiation of constructive dialogue. Social and political change seldom occurs in the absence of conflict. To the extent that these disagreements promote an increased awareness of the distinctive interests of disabled and nondisabled segments of society, they may be crucial to the continued emergence of a strong and unified international movement of people with disabilities.

SECTION FIVE: POLICY IMPLICATIONS

Vast changes are occuring in the development of policies and programs that affect persons with disabilities in many countries throughout the world. Although these measures express a widely accepted commitment to broad objectives such as increasing the employment of disabled individuals and improving their opportunities to enjoy a satisfactory and fulfilling life, they also contain varying assumptions and perspectives about the most effective means of achieving the goals. Moreover, these different approaches reflect distinct values which are the basic components of public policy. In a fundamental sense, normative concerns are inextricably interwoven with the analysis of efforts to solve pressing social problems. Since this investigation of European perceptions of attempts to promote the hiring of disabled workers has sought to examine important values embedded in laws and regulations concerning this subject, the research seems to encompass a corresponding obligation to assess the implications of these principles for the theory and practice of similar activities in the United States.

Perhaps the most critical issue in the study of the employment of disabled persons revolves about the definition of disability. In some European countries, vague or ambiguous standards, which were designed to reflect various conditions of the labor market, appeared to shape administrative practices that clouded the association between the distribution of resources and perceived needs. Similarly, although the research did not uncover any evidence that firms had engaged in a process of redefining the characteristics of employees in order to satisfy legal requirements, the use of relatively abstract criteria creates a potential for arguments about the danger of such abuse. In at least one nation, however, rigid definitions were regarded as overly technical and restrictive.

Many of the operational difficulties related to determinations of disability may have reflected basic weaknesses in the theoretical foundations upon which they were constructed. In Europe and the United States, programs to promote the employment of disabled citizens have been grounded on medical concepts of functional impairment and on definitions which incorporated assumptions about an industrial economy based on manual labor into public policy. Although a new approach to disability has been introduced by the enactment of American laws prohibiting discrimination against disabled individuals, this provision has not yet been adopted in European legislation. Yet many disabled persons in that region and elsewhere are beginning to perceive their problems primarily as the product of bias and segregation rather than as a consequence of personal restrictions or vocational limitations. For both political and administrative reasons, there appears to be a growing need to alter statutes and rules accordingly.

The formulation of public policy cannot be detached from the theoretical orientations and the research on which it is based. Perhaps one of the most serious deficiencies of existing approaches to disability—and to the development of pertinent legislation—is manifested by the relatively fragmented and disjointed themes which have dominated the discussion of this issue. Although some continuity has been found between medical and economic views of disability, each orientation reflects on essentially unidimensional understanding of the problems confronting disabled individuals. The life experiences of persons with disabilities are not confined to a preoccupation with their functional difficulties or to an exclusive concern with their tasks in the workplace. In fact, contrary to the expectations of many nondisabled observers, significant numbers of disabled people report that their lives are shaped more by the restraints which they encounter in a man-made environment and by the stigmatizing perceptions of other persons than by supposed inability to engage in common physical activities or by the demands of their occupational endeavors. In the world of the future, which can only be seen at a glimpse in the images of science fiction, human habitats may be adapted to the needs and requirements of each individual. Until that vision is realized, there seems to be a crucial need to reconceptualize the study of disability. Medical and economic concepts which comprise only a few dimensions of a person's life and which neglect the influence of the environment do not provide an adequate basis for comprehensive investigations of this subject. A disability is an attribute which permeates the lives of individuals who possess it. Research on disability must reflect a holistic perspective. Since success in resolving a major issue often is contingent upon a clear definition of the problem, this change also might yield significant improvements in the design of policies concerning disabled persons.

Prior efforts to create plans to promote the employment of people with disabilities usually have been dominated by professionals who are trained to provide assistance to disabled individuals. In fact, this focus has produced an impassive array of specialties including medicine, occupational therapy, physical therapy, special education, rehabilitation counseling, social work, gerontology, speech therapy, rehabilitation engineering, and others. Increasingly, this list is expanding to encompass law, architecture, urban planning, business or management, public administration, and similar fields which are beginning to recognize the crucial connection between their traditional concerns and the problems posed by disability. Each area of study has developed a separate theoretical framework and, to a large extent, a distinctive vocabulary for assessing this issue. Although many commentators have advocated the adoption of a ''team approach'' to overcome the inherent divisiveness spawned by the emergence of these disciplines, there appears to be one important element which is missing in this development. These professions tend to treat disabled persons as objects of investigation rather than as a valued source of information which can contribute to their knowledge and growth. None has attempted to compile or to analyze the accumulated experience or perceptions of people with disabilities as a basis for its academic endeavors. Like other phenomena, this pattern has important policy implications. Many disabled individuals in Europe and the United States complain that employment and other programs are developed for them rather than by them. The distinctive insights produced by extensive experience with a disability seldom are embodied in public policy, and organizations representing citizens with disabilities often are consigned to a relatively minor role in the decision-making process.

Perhaps a major responsibility for the remediation of this omission must be assumed by colleges and universities which undertake the task of preparing professionals for careers which entail extensive work with disabled persons. A curriculum focusing on the study of disability and society could be established as a multi-disciplinary activity to supplement and complement the education received by students in various academic fields. Although the study of public policy affecting disabled individuals might form an important component of this curriculum, other significant elements may focus on the distinctive experiences of people with disabilities and the values which they have in common. Disabled persons often appear to be exposed to different processes of socialization that may yield valuable perspectives which are not necessarily shared by their nondisabled counterparts. In fact, these experiences suggest the possible existence of a previously undetected culture, or subculture, of disability which could become an important source of mutual support for disabled people. Many citizens with disabilities are expressing increased dissatisfaction with the effort to adjust and accommodate to the demands of an unbending and frequently inhospitable environment; they are asking society to accept and adapt to their needs and interests. An enhanced awareness and appreciation of values derived from continuing personal experience with disability could be an important factor not only in the training of professionals but also in the formulation of public policy.

In contrast to prevailing medical and economic orientations, the socio-political view of disability focuses on the disabling effects of the environment rather than of individual characteristics. Unlike the former schools of thought, the latter perspective appears to permit the development of a theoretical framework for examining the values and experiences of disabled persons and for assessing their status as members of a minority group. In this study, a disability continuum based on visibility and permanence also is presented as a possible operations measure of the latter concept. Whereas the research traditions perpetuated by prior economic and medical definitions of disability do not appear to be consistent with an interpretation of the social and political movement of disabled citizens as striving to achieve the goal of increased equality, the socio-political approach seems congruent with this explanation. Moreover, all of these concepts apparently are compatible with a definition of disability which emphasizes the roles "expected" of an individual in a social environment. Since the policies of almost all societies seem to reflect normative expectations about a person's capacity to master the environment as a fundamental prerequisite to citizenship, the agenda of the disability movement—which extends beyond the mere adoption of impartial practices to a massive restructuring of supposedly permanent building and institutions—raises new and unfamiliar issues for political leaders. Medical and economic dimensions of disability simply represent two aspects of a larger multifaceted phenomenon. There appears to be an increasing need for definitional constructs which are broad enough to allow a recognition that the social and political struggles of people with disabilities seem to represent a continuing quest for equal rights.

The crucial nature of the linkage between definitions and the implementation of legislative programs can be illustrated by the American experience. Although the basic elements of disability policy in this country were contained in the Rehabilitation Act of 1920, there was scarcely any mention of the issue in the Social Security Act of 1935 in large measure because of the definitional difficulties encountered by the framers of the latter bill. Subsequently, the log-jam was broken by a Senate report in the 1940s which laid the groundwork for the passage of programs of Aid to the Permanently and Totally Disabled (that was later identified as Supplemental Security Income) and of Social Security Disability Insurance. The Senate definition, which emphasized the inability to engage in "substantial gainful activity," can be viewed as equating the concept of disability and the notion of unemployability. These policies have created a common experience in the lives of numerous disabled Americans. After they have completed their initial training and experienced difficulty in finding work due to job discrimination or other reasons, many are compelled to apply for income-maintenance assistance in order to sustain themselves. Then, after they have been officially labeled by a government agency as unable to engage in "substantial gainful activity," or essentially unemployable, they may be expected to participate in a program of vocational rehabilitation to prepare them for return to the labor force or the status of an employable person. Moreover, under regulations which exist in many states, if they complete such a program, they can only be trained for "entry level" employment, which in effect means that they may have to start all over again. Although the limitations of the present study precluded an examination of the relationship between employment and social welfare policies in European countries, similar inconsistencies probably could be found in the laws and regulations of other nations of the world.

There are several possible solutions to these problems. First, new definitions could be constructed to break the seemingly inexorable connection between disability and unemployability. The recognition that the difficulties confronting disabled persons in finding a job may result from employment discrimination rather than from functional impairments or work limitations seems to represent an important step in this direction. Second, rules could be altered to permit the establishment of rehabilitation programs designed to upgrade the skills of workers with disabilities, including those who become disabled relatively late in life, so that they move into supervisory or managegerial positions which usually require less menial or physical labor. Restrictions concerning "entry level" might be interpreted as reflecting a greater concern about the financial limits imposed on rehabilitation agencies than about the needs of disabled clients or the demands of the economy. Third, efforts could be made to develop a close liaison between the implementation of "affirmative action" plans and the activities of rehabilitation personnel. Although the European experience indicates that job placement programs and responsibility for the enforcement of antidiscrimination measures should not be assigned to the same agency, there seems to be no reason to prevent rehabilitation professionals from examining the extent to which employers are in compliance with these provisions and assisting them in the fulfillment of legal obligations. In fact, these duties might provide an instructive means of acquainting vocational counselors with the persistent patterns of discrimination encountered by people with disabilities.

Pehaps one of the major factors impeding the effectiveness of employment and other programs affecting disabled citizens is embodied in the concept of paternalism (Hahn, 1982; Hahn, 1983). Persons with disabilities commonly have been relegated by professionals and well-intended members of the public to a subordinate role which has prevented them from participating in the formulation of policy and from determining their own destinies. An important manifestation of this tendency is reflected by the administrative difficulties which frequently plague the implementation of laws designed for disabled people. Few elected representatives are willing to return to their constituents with the candid admission that they voted against measures to assist individuals with disabilities. Yet these plans usually require substantial expenditures. As a result, legislation concerning disabled persons often reflects vague objectives such as increased employment which allows political leaders to express their sympathy for this segment of the population and to delegate the task of accomplishing these goals with inadequate resources to bureaucrats in the executive branch of government. Attention is shifted thereby from the legislative arena to administrative forums which are less likely to attract publicity which could arouse public indignation or discontent. Insufficient funding and a lack of compliance with legal requirements to employ disabled workers are pervasive problems in the United States and in Europe. These difficulties do not necessarily discredit the principles upon which legislation is based. Yet there is a pressing need to focus increased emphasis and influence on administrative practices to insure that they fulfill these promises contained in the statutes approved by elected officials.

The formulation of disability policy also has been strongly affected by the nature of organizations concerned with this issue. Reflecting the imprint of the medical model, these groups usually have been organized around specific diseases or diagnostic categories in a fragmented pattern which tends to diminish the common interests and strengths of the disability community.

Moreover, they have been primarily involved in offering services to people with disabilities rather than in supporting their efforts to end discrimination and to achieve equal rights. An important distinction between "service providers" and advocates of "disability rights" appears to be emerging in Europe and the United States. Although the former organizations have tended to dominate prior discussion of disability-related issues and the development of policy, the latter movement is gradually beginning to assume a role of expanding importance. Both thrusts appear to offer complementary and effective means of securing major objectives such as increased employment for disabled citizens. Clearly, therefore, some method must be found to alter existing emphases on these approaches and to give the proponents of "disability rights" a position which is proportionate, if not parallel, to the emphasis on the provision of services.

The results of such a reallocation of effort and resources could have an important impact on employment policy regarding citizens with disabilities. Perhaps one of the most crucial differences between measures such as employer subsidies, vocational training, or rehabilitation programs and alternative plans including the quota system is the extent to which they rely upon persuasion or other means of achieving the stated goal. While the former programs focus on encouraging firms to recognize the value of disabled personnel, the latter proposal stresses mandatory methods to insure that employers fulfill their responsibilities. The policies also seem to imply a differential use of educational and legal mechanisms to secure increased employment for disabled persons which is related to the identification of a lack of information or discrimination as the major source of the problem. If employers are simply unaware of the potential capabilities of disabled workers, the answer seems to be education. If discrimination is the basic cause of unemployment among people with disabilities, however, instructional activities may be an inadequate and inappropriate remedy; legal requirements would seem to be justified and necessary.

The contrasts between these perspectives also reflect varying emphasis on individualistic and collective values. Whereas attempts to persuade employers to accept disabled job seekers concentrate primarily on individuals, compulsory approaches tend to assume that governments, acting on behalf of the society as a whole, must play a larger role in achieving this outcome. This relationship seems to provide an interpretation for the stress which private charities and voluntary organizations have traditionally placed on service providing activities. It may also contribute to an explanation of the differences between European and American attitudes toward the quota system. In the context of European understandings of the concept of equality, quotas reflect an effort to restore a relative state of equilibrium between the seemingly intrinsic disadvantages imposed on disabled citizens and the predominant advantages enjoyed by the nondisabled. The principle of quotas represents a more forceful approach to the employment of people with disabilities than programs based on encouragement or persuasion. Quotas are a powerful weapon against persistent patterns of job discrimination which can be enforced through appropriate administrative measures. As a result, employment quotas for disabled workers, including a system of levies or fines based on the price structure of goods and the competitive advantage available to employers in the private marketplace, might be recommended for inclusion in federal policy in the United States along with the strict enforcement of antidiscrimination laws. Perhaps the major readjustment which this change might require is an increased recognition that serious inequalities often result from the characteristics of the social structure rather than the attributes of individuals and that governments may have an obligation to redress this imbalance. The goal of equality for citizens with disabilities cannot be achieved without a willingness by the nondisabled majority to accept increased responsibility for the attainment of this objective. The expenditures necessary to create an environment which is accessible to everyone obviously exceed the resources of disabled individuals. Until elimination of the segregation and discrimination produced by man-made barriers can be guaranteed as a basic right of citizenship, the dream of freedom and equality may never be realized. Hence, consideration also must be given to the adoption in the United States of a disability allowance similar to the British proposal to offset the additional costs which disabled persons must incur in order to become full members of the society. The payment of this type of allowance to all disabled people, regardless of income, would represent not only an important acknowledgement of the discriminatory burdens imposed upon disabled people by an inaccessible environment but also an increased awareness that compensation for this expense is a duty which must be assumed by the entire community rather than by disabled individuals.

In many fundamental respects, the vast social changes required to provide equality to citizens with disabilities seem to exceed the goals proposed by prior social and political movements. Disabled people are seeking not only increased employment but also the right to participate in many other activities from which they have previously been excluded by environmental restraints. As a result, their aspirations seem to suggest the need for new approaches to the resolution of political controversies.

In the past, efforts to accommodate the desires of new or emerging political movements have been conducted in an atmosphere permeated by a concept of scarce resources and by assumptions that the eventual solution to almost all social problems could be found through a constant process of economic growth. This perspective also seemed to be based on the presumption that existing allocations of resources would remain essentially undisturbed and that additional revenues produced by an expansion of the economy would be used to provide incremental rewards for entrenched interests and to appease the demand of groups which had previously experienced significant deprivations. The approach seemed to be ideally suited to the needs of politicians. As long as the economic pie continued to expand, everyone appeared to be relatively satisfied. Disappointments could be readily assuaged by repeated references to the familiar refrain of economic limitations. Moreover, elected officials were not compelled to engage in the painful act of placating new participants in political contests by taking benefits away from more established forces. As a result, almost no significant attempts have been made in the history of American politics to enact redistributive policies which would withdraw resources from groups which have enjoyed comparative affluence and transfer them to disadvantaged segments of the population. The struggle to gain equality for people with disabilities appears to contain a potential for introducing some new and disturbing influences into the political process. Proposals for employment quotas, a disability allowance, and the construction of an accessible environment eventually may compel government leaders to shift their attention from distributive to redistributive policies. This transition could require a corresponding move from the individualistic notion of ''equality of opportunity'' to a concept of ''equal shares'' based on societal responsibility to fulfill fundamental social and economic conditions as a basic right of citizens. Yet significant social progress seldom is achieved without sacrifice. The goals expressed by the social and political movement of disabled persons might represent the ultimate test of America's commitment to the value of equality.

REFERENCES

Adams, A.S. (1976, January-February). Rehabilitation consumerism: Confrontation of communication and cooperation? *Journal of Rehabilitation*, *42*, 25.

Berkowitz, M., Johnson, W., and Murphy, E. (1976). *Public policy toward disability*. New York: Praeger.

Bowe, F. (1978). *Handicapping America: Barriers to disabled people*. New York: Harper and Row.

Bowe, F. (1980). *Rehabilitating America*. New York: Harper and Row.

Brehn, H., Howards, I., and Nagi, S. (1980). *Disability, from social problems to federal program*. New York: Praeger.

Carnes, G.D. (1979). *European rehabilitation service providers and programs*. East Lansing: University Rehabilitation, Michigan State University.

DeJong, G. (1983). Defining and implementing the independent living concept. In N. Crewe and I. Zola (Eds.), *Independent living for physically disabled people* (pp. 4-27). San Francisco, CA: Jossey-Bass.

Easton, D. (1971). *The political system: An inquiry into the state of political science* (2nd ed.). New York: Knopf.

Eisenberg, M.G., Griggins, C., and Duval, R.J. (1982). *Disabled people as second-class citizens*. New York: Springer Pub. Co.

Finkelstein, V. (1980). *Attitudes toward disabled people*. New York: World Rehabilitation Fund.

Gliedman, J., and Roth, W. (1980). *The unexpected minority: handicapped children in America*. New York: Harcourt, Brace, Jovanovich.

Hahn, H. (1982, July-August). Disablity and rehabilitation policy: Is paternalistic neglect really benign? *Public Administration Review, 73*, 385-389.

Hahn, H. (1983, March/April). Paternalism and public policy, *Society, 20*, 36-46.

Hartz, L. (1955). *The liberal tradition in America: An interpretation of American political thought since the revolution*. New York: Harcourt, Brace, Jovanovich.

Johnson, W.G. and Lambrinos, J. (1983, March/April). Employment discrimination. *Society, 20*, 47-50.

Kramer, R.M. (1981). *Voluntary agencies in the welfare state*. Berkeley: University of California Press.

Kulkarn, M.R. (1983). *Quota systems and the employment of the handicapped*. East Lansing, Michigan: University Center for International Rehabilitation.

Livingston, J.C. (1979). *Fair game?: Inequality and affirmative action*. San Francisco: W.H. Freeman.

Nagi, S. (1979). The concept and measurement of disability. In E. Berkowitz (Ed.), *Disability Policies and Government Programs* (pp. 1-15). New York: Praeger.

Nobel, J.H. Jr. (1982). Predicting future disaiblity and rehabilitation policies in the United States from northwestern European experience. In J. Rubin and V. LaPorte (Eds.), *Alternatives in rehabilitating the handicapped: A policy analysis* (pp. 189-214). New York: Human Sciences Press.

Osmond, H. and Seigler, M. (1974). *Models of madness, models of medicine*. New York: Macmillan.

Pan, E.L., Backer, T.E., and Vash, C.L. (Eds.). (1980-83). *Annual Review of Rehabilitation*. New York: Springer.

Purtilo, R. (1981). *Justice, liberty, compassion: 'Humane' health care and rehabilitation*. New York: World Rehabilitation Fund.

Reubens, B.G. (1970). *The hard-to-employ: European programs*. New York: Columbia University Press.

Ryan, W. (1971). *Blaming the victim* (1st ed.). New York: Pantheon Books.

Safilios-Rothschild, C. (1970). *The sociology and social psychology of disability and rehabilitation*. New York: Random House.

Scotte, R.A. (1981). *The making of blind men: A study of adult socialization*. New Brunswick, N.J.: Transaction Books. (originally published 1969).

Smith, R.T., and Gebert, A.J. (1981). Social policy issues in invalidity programs: Cross-national perspectives. In G.L. Albrecht (Ed.), *Cross-national rehabilitation policies: A sociological perspective* (pp. 123-156). Beverly Hills, CA: Sage Publications.

Stubbins, J. (1982). *The clinical attitude in rehabilitation*. New York: World Rehabilitation Fund.

Young, E.W.D. (Forthcoming 1984). *Societal provisions for the long-term needs of the disabled in Britain and Sweden relative to decision-making in new-born intensive care units*. World Rehabilitation Fund.

Zimmer, A.B. (1981). *Employing the handicapped: A practical compliance manual*. New York: AMACOM.

COMMENTARY
Mary Croxen, Open University, United Kingdom.

At a time of growing concern, on both sides of the Atlantic, to involve the 'consumer' in the decision-making process, to evolve participative procedures in policy-making and intervention particularly in the area of employment policy, an analysis of how European disabled people viewed existing employment policies should have been a welcome document. The World Rehabilitation Fund is to be congratulated on their farsightedness in commissioning such a study. The actual study, however, is a disappointment to me. It presents serious problems in a number of areas.

Essentially the piece vacillates between two approaches yet succeeds in neither. It is half-polemical, although not written in a polemical style. It is also, at times, written as if it is an academic research study yet fails to meet, I would argue, even minimum requirements for an acceptable research study of this kind. Furthermore, the arguments presented do not appear to have an internal coherence and consistency.

One would normally expect in writing a commentary of this kind to address the central issues in the argument presented and discuss those. It is perhaps a measure of the loose articulation of this document that it is no easy task to quarry out what the central argument is. Structural, stylistic and presentational features, which would normally receive secondary emphasis are of paramount importance here because they have obscured or failed to focus what are the vital elements.

The work is presented in five sections. It is at times difficult to establish what the real focus of each section is and how it relates to the ongoing argument. The discussion does seem to hover round the issue of the definition of disability, assessment, the quota scheme, legislation and policy and equality.

The definition issue receives, quite rightly, considerable prominence. A new definition of disability is provided which, it is claimed, is a socio-political definition. The familiar medical and economic definitions of disability are summarily dismissed and a new definition based on 'visibility' and 'permanence' presented as a 'socio-political' approach. This is supposed to represent a socio-political orientation in that it is argued that it is the way that others *perceive* the disabled person and the degree of permanence that they attribute to his/her condition that are the essential basis for prejudice and segregation. Hahn suggests a disability continuum between least visible disabilities to most visible with degree of discrimination related to this continuum in direct proportion. It is a simplistic formula which assumes 'visibility' as a unitary characteristic (yet 'economic' definitions have just been dismissed as too 'undimensional' in character) and similarly 'discrimination' as having some sufficiently homogenous qualities to put forward such a linear equation. Even a quadratic equation would not do, however, as the argument contains some profoundly blind assumptions and most seriously of all sets back thinking about disability by a decade. Masquerading as a 'socio-political' definition, veneered with stylish intellectual prose is a definition which locates disability unquestionably *in* the person not in the relationships of which he is a part. The mutual responsibility and dynamic aspects of relationships are missing…One winces to read…"Although primary emphasis is placed on physical characteristics which may *trigger* prejudice and discrimination…" It is not surprising given the implicit location of the problem *in* the client (stated as how he is perceived but nevertheless based on his/her presenting characteristics) that a quota system which is a 'segregated' route into integrated employment should be chosen for these people. It is, in my view, a wholly lamentable position. Mentally handicapped people although squeezed into the formula do not receive adequate consideration.

The paper presents further difficulties, however, Hahn is himself one of the *disabled consumers* in the United States and, I would think, is *known to be so*. One would expect therefore very much of an 'inside' view: a view of confederates. It is indeed a view of confederates but not of the kind we might have expected. Hahn has mingled with the mighty in the disabled community and has presented the views of the *European disabled elite*—doubly elite because not only have they risen to the top of their own organisations as spokespersons, but also have not experienced the usual educational limitations of a career in disability provides in that they were often linguistically competent enough to speak to Hahn in his own native language rather than their own. The views therefore are of a coterie of disabled intellectuals—people who have not necessarily drunk to the dregs the bitter cup of failure to make it on the labour market. One senses, however, that Hahn is not even part of this privileged group, but is on the outside—a political scientist seeking grist to his mill or pillaging conversations which illustrate his own predetermined view. This is not necessarily how disabled people feel in Europe about employment policies, but *a collage of views* which texture and colour in Hahn's poorly directed argument. Frequently spokespersons from all four countries are put together as a collective 'European' view. Sometimes when the 'European' perspective is given it seems as if rehabilitation professionals, government officials, voluntary organisations and organisations of disabled people are put together to form one constituency. This really will not do. This purports to be representative of European views. It is unfortunately, not clear who the 'spokespersons' are, how they were selected, what they were asked or what their understanding of the study in question was. We are not told about the selection strategy as regards the interviews, no details of the 'in depth' interviews. It is difficult without some indication of the source of the quotations to evaluate them. Issues of confidentiality one would have thought would only be of concern to those who were in the government service. There does not seem to have been an attempt to collate comprehensibly the material collected. The bibliography of the work is consistent with my view that it does not reflect European views. The listed publications are all from American publishing houses—the only U.K. reference (Massie) is missing from the list. Some of the difficulties of establishing European 'views' on employment policy might have been ameliorated by a more extensive reading of literature emanating from the four countries in question. I accept that many of the works cited are indeed overviews of European work. I would have felt more confident, however, had some original sources been consulted.

The monograph presents further problems in its discussion of the quota system in the U.K., F.R.G. and France. There is no clear statement of what these schemes are in each of these countries and there is the implication that comparisons are being made of like with like. This is not the case. The quota scheme in the United Kingdom is targeted on a much wider group than that of the F.R.G. The differences between providing employment for people who would in no other way find employment on the open labour market by means of a quota and a levy scheme as in Germany and the attempts to provide employment to a much wider category of disabled people as in the United Kingdom System are not directly comparable in the way implied. The inclination to treat quota systems in a homogenous way evidenced in this report means that the systems themselves are seriously misrepresented.

M. C.

COMMENTARY ON: THE ISSUE OF EQUALITY: EUROPEAN PERCEPTIONS OF EMPLOYMENT POLICY FOR DISABLED PERSONS by Harlan Hahn and COMMENTARY by Mary Croxen

Joseph Stubbins, California State University, Los Angeles.

The prevailing professional view of unemployment is that disabled persons lack an adequate appraisal of their assets and liabilities, need vocational training, skill in presenting themselves and so on; in short, the answer is clinical assessment and counseling to make them more competitive in the labor market and to place them in jobs. Hahn's perspective as a political scientist is a refreshing departure from these familiar paths of vocational rehabilitation and gives proper importance to the structural features of society by which disabled persons are handicapped in the labor market. His socio-political views open up many possibilities for theorizing and practice that are new for the field of vocational rehabilitation.

Hahn's theory is that the most productive way of conceptualizing the second-class status of disabled persons is to regard them as members of a disadvantaged group comparable to certain ethnic groups. They are subject to the same kind of stereotyping and discrimination. To one degree or another members of disadvantaged groups tend to interiorize the negative views which dominant groups have of them. Therefore, Hahn places great importance on group organization for the purpose of consciousness raising. That is viewed as preliminary to political activism.

He develops his views by comparing employment policies for disabled people in four European countries and the United States. In each country, he interviewed representatives of grassroots organizations, traditional organizations for the disabled and government officials. His observations are couched in general terms so that one does not learn much detail about prevailing employment practices (which could differ from expectations based on policies). On brief contacts of the kind Hahn had, it is easy to come away with misconceptions of what happens in the field. However, there is so little discussion in the United States concerning disability policies and practices in other industrialized countries that this monograph would be welcomed by those who foresee the values of cross-national exchange of rehabilitation ideas.

Attempts to interest American rehabilitation professionals in considering, for instance, the quota system are most frequently met with, ''It wouldn't work in the USA.'' Hahn has rendered a useful service by normalizing the differences in employment policies among countries by relating them to different notions of equality and other cultural dimensions. Most of our welfare policies emerged later than in Europe and many were modeled after European ones—a lesson of history that is not widely known. Presumably Hahn gained some inspiration from what he learned abroad that would prove useful in the U.S. or result in cultural change. At any rate, he apparently approached his European experience with pretty strong convictions which is clear from the first part of the monograph.

What I found most positive about Hahn's monograph is that it deals with disability policies in generic terms and at the national level. In relation to the vast sums spent on income maintainence and rehabilitation for disabled persons and the enormous changes in technology which make them available for work, there is meager attention to the need for policy review of the whole gamut of handicapped legislation. At present we have a complex agglomeration of programs based on outmoded concepts of disability and the fortunes of political constituencies. It is rare for such issues to be brought into focus.

In view of the new ground Hahn has ploughed, the monograph's shortcomings are unfortunate. If the positivism underlying traditional vocational rehabilitation suffers from the analysis of the individual divorced from social and structural context, Hahn has erred in the opposite direction by unsuccessfully incorporating too much in a single monograph. Those parts which dealt directly with the issue of equality, I found interesting and helpful. Some parts I could only relate to with difficulty. For example, the extensive discussion of definitions of disability, important though it is, could have been integrated with his policy discussion.

The importance Hahn attached to the visibility and permanency of a disability and their relation to discrimination was not evident to me. I know of no empirical evidence to support this hypothesis but some to refute it. In any event, ''visibility'' and ''permanency'' are ambiguous terms as he presented them.

Hahn's writing style puts a burden on the reader. Academics are socialized into writing for their peers who are accustomed to abstractions which become a familiar language to the in-group. Since social scientists often deal with subjects about which most citizens have strong opinions, they tend to buttress their expertise with stodgy expressions which become habitual. Many career rehabilitation readers might think it presumptuous for an outsider (a political scientist) to have opinions about what transpires on their turf. Therefore, the shortcomings noted above would make it too easy to discount the essential value of Hahn's attempt to interpret disability in social and political terms.

Clearly, there are some similarities between the above commentary and Croxen's. However, there are striking differences. I will try to account for these as cultural phenomena in the light of my experience in the United Kingdom during 1979—1980 (Stubbins, 1982) as well as other experiences abroad. Because of our common language and somewhat similar institutions, there is a tendency to under-estimate our differences.

In the U.K., persons with a broad liberal education from one of the universities (rather than the polytechnic institutions) are usually preferred for leadership posts over what Americans would consider better qualified technically trained persons. For instance, I encountered only one person in a senior position in the Resettlement Service of the Manpower Services Commission who came up through the ranks; the others came in directly to their posts without technical or practical experience. This cultured gentleman concept of the good leader contrasts with American distrust of intellectuals and emphasis on technical training. Now what does this have to do with the different perceptions of Hahn's monograph by a British and American critic?

By British standards, probably Hahn's monograph would be judged more stringently than by American ones—partly, because an educated Briton considers what he wrote a measure of himself and partly because the American rehabilitation scene is not understood.

About writing style: The prevailing American pragmatic attitude tends to view a document much more in terms of its utility than its style or elegance. It is rare for a British Resettlement Officer to write an article about his rehabilitation experience presumably because he or she felt it would not be published. Yet they are the only ones in the government service with line experience and their collective wisdom was poorly exploited by senior government officials. I am satisfied to relate to those parts of Hahn's paper that serve the interests of disabled persons and put the others in the background.

About the American rehabilitation scene: Croxen evidently is not in touch with the intellectual climate in which American rehabilitation is embedded. Her British background and familiarity with Common Market countries are, so to speak, handicapping in understanding the ideology which undergirds rehabilitation here. Marxism and structuralism are much more familiar to British academics than to their American counterparts. Therefore, Hahn's advocacy of socio-political perspectives on disability is hardly news to Croxen. Conceivably she finds it hard to visualize that in the U.S. Hahn's approach to employment policies for the disabled would encounter great resistance here.

REFERENCES

Stubbins, J. (1982) *The clinical attitude in rehabilitation: A cross-cultural view.* New York: World Rehabilitation Fund.

I suppose that I should be grateful to Mary Croxen. During the past several years, in addressing rehabilitation professionals and other predominantly nondisabled audiences, I have sometimes wished that I had an opponent. Frequently I have sensed that my views concerning the social and political movement to secure equal rights for disabled persons had been courteously received but just as politely ignored. The paternalistic attitudes that commonly permeate relationships between nondisabled and disabled people have seemed to obscure real and meaningful differences of opinion. In attempting to display sympathetic agreement with the goals of disabled citizens, others have been reluctant to admit—consciously or publicly—that the eventual implications of this movement might impinge on their own professional or political interests. Too often, rehabilitation personnel as well as other nondisabled observers have focused almost exclusively on efforts to reduce the vocational and functional effects of a disability, persons with disabilities have emphasized policies designed to eliminate prejudice and discrimination, and there has been relatively little constructive dialogue between the two groups about these contrasting approaches. Croxen has candidly recorded her apparently implacable disagreement with my work, and I can only hope that the controversy which could be generated by her vehement criticism might prompt additional readers to examine my ideas carefully in an expanded search for a solution to the employment and other problems confronting people with disabilities throughout the world.

I would be less than honest, however, if I did not also express the wish that her commentary had been somewhat less personal and vitriolic. I find it psychologically painful to read such relentlessly negative and hostile criticism from a colleague whom I have respected. It is especially distressing to see my ethics impugned with accusations that I have conducted "embarassingly poor research" and that I have engaged in "pillaging conversations" to fit my "predetermined view." Such reckless charges cannot destroy my reputation or integrity as a researcher. Anyone who chooses to do so is welcome to examine my scholarly career and academic record of almost twenty years before I embarked on the study of disability and rehabilitation policy. However damaging these personal attacks may prove to be, I would prefer to focus this discussion on other issues.

Croxen does not merely challenge my capabilities and methods as a social scientist, she does not like what I have to say. The customary mild acceptance of a few thoughts, at least, which ordinarily lends balance even to the fiercest intellectual criticism, is conspicuously lacking from her commentary. Apparently, she has found the work devoid of any redeeming features whatsoever. Ironically, however, her critique scarcely mentions the major concepts such as equality and civil rights which I sought to present.

The responsibility of securing acceptance for such ideas now seems even more crucial than the task of preparing them for dissemination. For, if Croxen is successful in planting doubts about the value of the concepts after they have appeared in print, there is a grave danger that they might be subsequently discounted. And, if these ideas are dismissed because of her criticism, they could be relegated to the same status of benign neglect which might not otherwise have been their fate. Some casual readers (and others who learn about the monograph without reading it) may be tempted to say, "Oh, Croxen refuted those theories anyway." I suggest that this judgment is not only untrue, but it would also represent a critical mistake. The thoughts which I have tried to make available in this work might be inadequately phrased, or they may have been stated more effectively by others; but the concepts are of great importance. Ideas such as equality and civil rights should not be discredited by unsubstantiated assertions or intemperate expressions of displeasure.

In an odd way, Croxen's objections are both extraordinarily intense and exceptionally abstract. The work is characterized as "a disappointment," which lacks "internal coherence and consistency" and "central issues" as well as "direction, structure, and a proper evaluation," and reflecting a "poorly directed argument." Yet the reader may search in vain for a specific point, remark, or idea to which these pejorative labels are attached. Although she complains that there is not "some breathtaking denouement at the end of the document," for example, she does not directly contest any of the major conclusions or policy recommendations. Significantly, even though Coxen's commentary does not appear to include a single positive statement about the concepts expressed in the monograph, there is also no detailed criticism of any of the substantive ideas contained therein. The paradox prompted me to seek an explanation for the fury of Croxen's response. What could possibly be so threatening as to stimulate such an intense reaction? In retrospect, I recognize that I may have made a mistake. The concepts of equality and civil rights which I sought to develop on the basis of a sociopolitical definition of disability do not represent a minor modification or addendum to the theoretical frameworks which have traditionally guided rehabilitation as well as other disability-related disciplines. Fundamentally, they comprise the foundations of an alternative paradigm. This admission may contribute to an explanation of the amorphous but severe nature of the criticism directed at my analysis. At the very least, it helps me understand why, in reading Croxen's comments for the first time, I felt like an infidel accused of heresy in a searing inquisition. I guess that some of my ideas might appear heretical. They do seem to reflect a departure from orthodox viewpoints in rehabilitation. Perhaps, in more ways than I imagined at the time I first committed them to paper, the concepts represent a challenge to established modes of thinking in disability-related professions. The conflict over my work cannot be interpreted as a dispute concerning research methods or appropriate means of organizing information. Fundamentally, it constitutes an apparently unavoidable collision of substantive ideas. Neither the diffuse nature of the critique nor my own desire to secure a favorable reception for the concepts should be allowed to conceal the tension between conventional models of rehabilitation and approaches founded on the principles of equality and civil rights. There are essential subjects about which Croxen and I simply seem to disagree.

Perhaps some additional background about my perspective is in order. For several years, I have developed an increasing belief that there is an urgent need to reconceptualize the study of disability. This position was born more than five years ago when, during a sabbatical from my university, I conducted a broad survey of the literature on disability and rehabilitation policy. The effort not only exposed me to an unusually fragmented and disjointed body of research, but it also produced a realization that few of the available studies seemed to bear any relation to my own experience as a disabled person. In an effort to learn more, I enrolled at another nearby university and earned a master's degree in rehabilitation counseling. This training, which I found highly valuable, also led me to recognize that most of the assumptions, conceptual approaches, and theoretical orientations in rehabilitation were not closely related to what I regard as the most crucial problems confronting people with disabilities. This conviction was strengthened and reinforced by numerous discussions with disabled individuals in the United States and Europe. In many respects, this monograph reflects the manner in which my thinking has evolved on the basis of these visits. *Even though we did not always share a similar verbal or signing linguistic tradition, I soon discovered that we did speak the same language. Our communication and understanding were based on our common experience as persons with disabilities.*

Large numbers of disabled people have become part of an expanding social and political movement which has far-ranging implications for rehabilitation and other professions. Increasingly, disabled citizens may begin to demand equal treatment in employment decisions as a civic right rather than as a practice requiring extraordinary incentives, preparation, modifications, persuasion, or placement activities. In a society environmentally designed to ensure equality between disabled and nondisabled residents, there might be a reduced need for rehabilitation or other special programs. This prospect is apt to produce ambivalent feelings among professionals providing services to disabled individuals. Many might deny the possibility of such a society, and some may argue that it still would not solve unemployment and other problems facing disabled people. Yet most probably would acknowledge that slow progress is being made in this direction, and few would openly dispute the legitimacy of the goal of genuine equality in an environment fully adapted to the needs of disabled and nondisabled citizens. The strain between this objective and the traditional aim of rehabilitation is at the center of the controversy.

Whereas conventional rehabilitation practices view improvements in the functional and occupational capacities of disabled individuals as an almost exclusive means of reducing unemployment among this segment of the population, the disability rights movement focuses on eradicating bias and discrimination as the primary solution. As long as the divergent implications of these two perspectives remain unexplored, communications between these groups is likely to be fraught with discord.

Mounting awareness of the apparent discrepancy between these orientations seemed to dictate the preparation of the analysis. From the marvelous vantage point of hindsight, I believe that my principal fault was to permit the contradictions between these approaches to remain implicit rather than making them explicit. My work focused on employment policies for disabled persons in Europe and especially the principle of quotas, which is the major feature differentiating European and American programs. Yet there seemed to be a basic incompatibility between the investigation of this subject and existing assumptions and perspectives in rehabilitation. Clearly, if rehabilitation were optimally successful in improving the vocational and functional capabilities of disabled persons, and if this comprised an adequate solution to employment problems, there would be little need for quotas, antidiscrimination laws, or similar measures. The fact that the former approach has not been conspicuously successful is indicated by extraordinarily high rates of unemployment among disabled people everywhere. Most rehabilitation professionals have responded to this situation by intensifying their attempts to achieve even further improvements in the functional and work skills of disabled individuals. Imbued with the anticipation that the traditional theory and practice of rehabilitation will eventually lead to a solution to the problem, they have been understandably reluctant to pursue alternative avenues. Perhaps this expectation also explains why the analysis of major provisions of disability policy such as quotas has usually been consigned to the periphery of rehabilitation research. The examination of policy issues should not be regarded as an unwelcome distraction from the usual concerns of this discipline.

In order to provide a foundation for this work, therefore, it was necessary to introduce a new theoretical perspective. The major components of this approach were represented by a socio-political definition of disability, by an investigation of American and European understandings of the concept of equality, and by the views of the emerging international social and political movement of disabled persons. The development of this alternative paradigm was deemed essential not only to form an adequate framework for the analysis of the principle of quotas in employment policy but also to alter some of the beliefs which have dominated the field of rehabilitation for many years. The attainment of the former goal seemed dependent on the latter effort. Yet, in pursuing this aim, I may have neglected to make my purpose and my disagreements with prevailing assumptions as clear as possible. I should be pleased to have the opportunity to do so now. I am compelled to state, after careful study and an extensive review of the literature, that there appears to be a deep gulf between conceptual interests which previously shaped the field of rehabilitation and the policy issues which are the primary focus of this analysis. I further believe that this incongruity has contributed to the nonenforcement of quotas, affirmative action requirements, and other laws to prohibit discrimination against disabled workers. I am also convinced that there is a pressing need to reconceptualize disability so that these crucial subjects can be brought within the purview of rehabilitation and similar disciplines. My work is consciously designed to permit and to facilitate this development.

The explanation comprises necessary background which also allows a direct response to Croxen's diffuse and sweeping charges. The "central issues" of the analysis should be abundantly clear by now. The core of the work is embodied by concepts of equality and civil rights and by policy proposals such as quotas which might contribute to their fulfillment by combatting employment discrimination. Although prior studies in rehabilitation have tended to exclude these matters, the theme was deliberately chosen in the hope that it would guide subsequent research in this field. In addition, the comments should help to clarify Croxen's apparent confusion about the so-called "polemical" or scholarly nature of the analysis. Strictly speaking, of course, the work is not polemics. It is admittedly designed to stimulate changes in the traditional theoretical paradigm of rehabilitation by advancing concepts which have been previously neglected or ignored. Many of these ideas also have been put forward by the international social and political movement of disabled persons. This conjunction, however, should not be interpreted as reflecting narrowly partisan purposes. On the contrary, the dominant paradigms of many academic disciplines have been altered by trends and perspectives which have emerged elsewhere. To contend that scholarly investigations should remain impervious to such developments would be almost tantamount to arguing that existing theoretical frameworks are completely neutral or value-free. Most researchers increasingly acknowledge that widely accepted theories usually reflect normative concerns. The task of the analyst, therefore, is to ferret out the paradigmatic restrictions which seem to preclude or foreclose appropriate areas of inquiry and to introduce concepts that appear to meet perceived needs or the legitimate aspirations of important actors outside the ordinary confines of the professional community.

Although Croxen's supposed quandary about whether to call my analysis "polemics" or "an academic research study" seemed to prevent the recognition of ts actual purpose as an effort to change a dominant paradigm, she nonetheless proceeds to assess it as a conventional empirical study and to subject it to scorching criticism on that basis. Since she has missed this point in the analysis, the critique is not as relevant as it might otherwise have been. Yet, the charges do deserve a reply and an explanation.

Croxen concentrates relentlessly on the selection of the persons whom I visited in Europe. Her criticism ignores the fact that, since there is no universe of European leaders of organizations of disabled citizens or other observers, samplng procedures are impossible and meaningless. She even apparently wants to know whom I have quoted and argues that "confidentiality" should not be a bar to the disclosure of my sources. But I promised the informants anonymity, and I cannot renege on that promise. Croxen chastises me for not including "emphatic disclaimers" that the informants cannot be considered "representative." But I did not claim that they were representative; and, most importantly, the issue of representativeness is irrelevant to the merit of their views. This is qualitative field research. Resources were not available for the sort of quantitative research which Croxen is criticizing. Qualitative field investigations may not be as familiar as other types of research, but this does not invalidate the inquiry. If Croxen or others wish to assess its reliability, I would welcome such an endeavor. The results of my effort, which I sought to report as fully as possible, yielded an extraordinarily rich and meaningful body of information, insights, opinions, suggestions, and recommendations. I find it difficult to imagine how it would be possible to improve on the quality of these *perceptions*. In the type of investigation which I was pursuing, attention must be directed at an appraisal of the value of the ideas which were uncovered. Croxen's unwillingness to evaluate the analysis by standards which are appropriate to this kind of research suggests that she is not only concerned about methods but also about the substantive ideas contained in this work and in the views expressed by the observers whom I visited.

A confusion of methodological and theoretical issues also seems to pervade Croxen's derisive comments about the bibliography. She makes the elementary mistake of assuming that I have not consulted the European publications which I did not cite. I suppose that I could have "padded" the references by including these books, but little would be gained by such an exercise. Although I have done an extensive amount of reading in European sources, I generally found them devoid of innovative perspectives which might contribute to the analysis of the concept of quotas or to the development of an alternative theoretical paradigm in rehabilitation. Like many of the informants who expressed original and creative ideas about employment policies affecting disabled persons, I was seeking a new approach to the examination of these subjects. Referring repeatedly to familiar but outmoded sources would not have added to this endeavor.

There are also major inconsistencies in Croxen's comments about the organization of the analysis. She claims that issues "come in and out of focus." She charges that I have not made "an attempt to collate comprehensibly the material collected." And yet she asserts that there are "no details of the 'in depth' interviews." I have made a major effort to report accurately and completely what I was told during the interviews in Europe. This practice follows the accepted canons of qualitative field research. Although occasional commentary was necessary to preserve the flow of the analysis, I did not try to fit these views into a Procrustean mold. I sought to allow the informants to speak for themselves. And still their opinions are dismissed as "a collage of views which texture and colour in Hahn's...argument." Perhaps there might have been more organization or less organization of the information from the interviews but it would be impossible to satisfy both demands simultaneously. In rereading section four, I would now conclude that I erred on the side of too much "detail." But if I had attempted to impose more structure upon this material, I might have been exposed not ony to the risk of transgressing the standards of this type of anlysis but also to the accusation that I had manipulated the presentation to suit my so-called "predetermined view." I would prefer to let these data stand. For those who wish to examine carefully the viewpoints which I have reported, there are some vitally important ideas to be gleaned from this section. For the more casual reader, summaries are available. But there appears to be no means of mollifying all of Croxen's strident objections. The contradictions in her criticism only seem to reaffirm the impression that she is more concerned about the content than the organization of this information.

Ironically, after stating these complaints, Croxen proceeds to demand more specifics about the quota system in the United Kingdom, the Federal Republic of Germany, and France. At first blush, her suggestion "to have this detailed information in...an appendix" seemed appealling. Although most of these facts are contained in Kulkarni (1983) and other readily available sources, I was prepared to do any additional work which might be required to assist the reader in following the analysis. And yet I gradually realized that the inclusion of such an appendix would not only complicate rather than simplify the presentation, but it would also detract from a major focus of the work. *This analysis has sought to confine the discussion of quotas to perceptions of the principle which they reflect. It is not intended to be an exhaustive or definitive examination of the operation of the quota system in each of the three countries.* Throughout the analysis, I have attempted to draw a clear distinction between the concept of a quota and its implementation. This emphasis does not "seriously misrepresent" the nature of quotas. The approach is consistent with the widely accepted dichotomy between political issues and administrative questions. In fact, a central conclusion of this work is that the administrative reluctance to enforce quotas does not diminish their value as a means of gaining employment for disabled workers. Thus, to present additional details about the complexity of the quota system would be both premature and inconsistent with this investigation. For many years, European quotas have been discounted because of widespread noncompliance with their provisions. Mixing conceptual issues and administrative difficulties again would only tend to perpetuate the myth that the principle of quotas is hopelessly ineffective. *This investigation has disclosed qualitatively significant support for the concept of quotas, especially among leaders of organizations of disabled citizens*, and it has reported some excellent suggestions which were proposed to increase their practical clout. The examination of the detailed provisions of the quota system in different countries would seem to be an especially appropriate topic for further study.

In this response to Croxen's commentary, I have attempted to make it clear that our real disagreement does not revolve around different research methods, standards, or any of the other issues that ostensibly shape academic criticism. Fundamentally our contrasting positions stem from divergent social values. Nowhere is this source of conflict more evident than in her criticisms of quotas and the socio-political definition of disability. Croxen does not support my approach, theories, or findings because she does not appear to agree with this definition of disability which is basic to the work. In a crucial respect, the outcome could not have been otherwise. The socio-political definition is an essential foundation for the analysis that follows. Disagreement with this conceptualization is almost certain to yield oppositon to the subsequent investigation. Perhaps Croxen's commentary could have been more coherently organized if she had concentrated on definitional issues rather than scattering hyperboles so widely. Nevertheless, I welcome the opportunity to join the controversy at this level.

Although Croxen apparently prefers the "familiar" medical and economic definitions of disability to the socio-political approach, the real ground of her objections to the latter concept are not immediately apparent. She does attack the disability continuum, which is based on the socio-political perspective, as "simplistic" presumably because she believes it assumes that visibility is a "unitary characteristic." (In reply, I can only say that, while I agree that many phenomena impinge on human perceptions, I believe their salience shrinks in comparison with the crucial distinction between visibility and invisibility.) She also claims that discrimination does not have "homogeneous qualities." I will have more to say about that later. Nonetheless, on the basis of these brief assertions, she concludes that "the argument contains some profoundly blind assumptions" and, "most seriously," that I have "set back thinking about disability by a decade." This is, indeed, a serious accusation. If I believed for a moment that there was any substance to it whatsoever, I would certainly withdraw my work from publication and quietly retreat from the study of disability, never to be heard from again. However, I must emphatically reject this astonishing and audacious allegation. I have merely sought to bring the discussion of disability up to date with concepts contained in legislation of the nineteen-seventies. *I am convinced that modern perspectives will increasingly acknowledge that disability can be found primarily in a disabling environment rather than in the individual.* The contrast between Croxen's position and my own view is displayed most clearly on this issue. The difference reflects competing theoretical orientations. I suspect that many readers supporting Croxen's judgment will be those who are so passionately and exclusively devoted to the goal of improving the functional and occupational capacities of disabled people that they are unwilling to consider alternative approaches. By contrast, I predict that others may respond by recognizing that I have attempted to develop a perspective which permits the analysis of discrimination and inequality as major problems confronting people with disabilities. I leave it to others to decide whether my ideas represent progress or the opposite.

Croxen's attempt to concentrate attention on "presenting characteristics" rather than on "perceptions" not only reflects a crucial misrepresentation of my analysis, but it also illustrates the wide discrepancy between our positions. The meaning which Croxen has tried to impute to the socio-political perspective is more compatible with the traditional rehabilitation focus on improving the functional and vocational skills of the disabled individual than with the effort to end bias and discrimination. The goals of the former approach seem to reflect a desire to minimize the effects of disability so that they might eventually be rendered almost imperceptible. The purpose of the latter perspective is to change the environment and the behavior of others rather than to seek infinite improvements in the person with a disability. These objectives are not easily reconcilable, but they should not be clouded by misstatements or misapprehensions.

Perhaps one of the most basic factors underlying Croxen's criticism of this analysis is her opposition to quotas for disabled workers. She reproaches me for endorsing quotas, which she characterizes as "a 'segregated' route into integrated employment...for these people." It is, according to her, "a wholly lamentable position." Such strong language again must not be allowed to conceal the unspoken assumption in her objection. Croxen displays an extreme dislike for a separate approach to the hiring of disabled persons. Her view is consistent with the conventional emphasis on improving functional and vocational capabilities to meet the standards prescribed by and for nondisabled people. By contrast, I find exclusion from employment and from many other common activities a pervasive fact of life for most disabled citizens. Segregation cannot be eradicated by pretending it does not exist. The classification implied by the principle of quotas simply reflects the reality that disabled and nondisabled job seekers are treated differently in the labor market. Moreover, combined with adequate administrative mechanisms to secure compliance, quotas comprise an especially appropriate device for eradicating discrimination. There is nothing inherently "lamentable" about quotas when they are employed as a tool to gain access for members of groups which have been previously excluded from major social and economic structures rather than as a restriction on the number of these individuals admitted to such institutions. I admit that the prospect of securing approval for the principle of quotas in a country such as America, which has embraced traditions of individualism and equality of opportunity, is, as I have indicated, an uphill fight. Yet the insights expressed by the European observers whom I visited, and especially the leaders of organizations of disabled citizens, seem to offer a persuasive case for the consideration of a strengthened quota plan, with effective enforcement provisions, as a viable means of combatting unemployment and discrimination.

What, then, is the seemingly irreconcilable cleavage between Croxen's view and my position? A major part of the answer can be ascribed to the contrast between the traditional rehabilitation paradigm and the socio-political perspective. Another portion probably can be attributed to a difference of opinion about definitions, the concept of discrimination, and the principle of quotas. In addition, however, Croxen seems to imply that there are other sources of disagreement.

Croxen ostensibly attributes her disappointment with the results of this investigation to the allegation that I have "presented the views of the European disabled elite." She then attempts to discount their ideas by claiming that they are the opinions of "a coterie of disabled intellectuals—people who have not necessarily drunk to the dregs the bitter cup of failure to make it on the labour market." There are several statements which must be made in response to this portion of her attack.

First, the persons whom I visited in Europe were not members of an "elite." Many of the disabled leaders were underemployed, and some were unemployed. Few were wealthy or even financially comfortable. Hardly any of them enjoyed significant social or political influence in their societies. Many discussions also were conducted with the kind assistance of an interpreter. Yet, as the statements quoted in this work demonstrate, these disabled Europeans possessed a rare ability to analyze complex policy issues.

Second, even if this group were branded an "elite," the label does not invalidate the inquiry. A foreign observer interested in new rehabilitation techniques in the United Kingdom would not be compelled to interview every DRO or even a cross-section of them. A physician wanting to learn about advanced medical procedures in Sweden would not be expected to visit ordinary practitioners in that country. Their attention might naturally be focused on leaders in the field. Representativeness is neither implied nor required in the type of qualitative field investigation which I conducted. Although the leaders of European organizations of disabled citizens comprise the group whose opinions have been most often ignored in previous discussions of quotas and other aspects of disability policy, there is no reason to impose restrictions on this analysis which would not be applied to the study of other groups or issues.

Third, people with disabilities may have opinions on policy issues which transcend supposed distinctions between ''elites'' and ''masses.'' Attempts to dismiss the views of disabled leaders or ''intellectuals'' by superimposing such a dualism upon this segment of the population might neglect the common experiences and values shared by all disabled persons. Perhaps rehabilitation personnel are accustomed to hearing sincere expressions of gratitude for the services they provide disabled ''consumers'' in an otherwise inhospitable environment. Job discrimination, however, is a prevalent and continuing problem for many employed and unemployed disabled people who have drunk numerous bitter cups of failure in the labor market. Nondisabled professionals could profit from increased knowledge of the social and political attitudes of citizens with disabilities.

Perhaps Croxen and other nondisabled observers seem to be unaware of the implications of the emerging international social and political movement of disabled persons. This trend is hardly mentioned in her commentary. Admittedly, there has been little coverage of this subject either in the mass media or in professional rehabilitation journals. Research funding to examine the scope or extent of this development also has been generally unavailable. And yet the demand for equal rights, which is a basic tenet of this movement, has been expressed not only by leaders of organizations of disabled citizens throughout the world but also by other segments of the disabled population. In fact, a major informal discovery of my fellowship study-visit was the extent to which the principles of the disability rights movement in the United States were known, respected, and endorsed by disabled Europeans. Among the latter group, such ideas usually implied support for the concept of quotas. These may not have been the perceptions which Croxen wanted or expected to find, but they reflect a growing sentiment which rehabilitation personnel can ignore only at the risk of perpetuating a potentially serious misunderstanding.

Despite her naivete about the subject, Croxen is determined to convince the reader that this analysis ''is not necessarily how disabled people feel in Europe about employment policies.'' That her pursuit of this aim apparently knows no bounds is demonstrated by her charge that I am ''not even part'' of the group of disabled pesons whom I visited. According to her, I am ''on the outside—a political scientist seeking grist to his mill.'' This is a highly personal attack; and, in spite of my reluctance to discuss such issues, I cannot disregard it. It is despicable and insulting. She seems to be trying to cast me outside the disability community. Apparently she feels that she is not only an expert on the attitudes of people with disabilities but also that she has the power to expel me from a movement with which she herself is not familiar. Such dazzling audacity is beyond belief. I leave it to the leaders of the disability rights movement to decide whether I am inside or outside this community. And I submit that they are the only persons capable of making that determination. People with disabilities are quite tired of having others tell them what they think and who their spokespersons should be. Such efforts bear a close resemblance to the smugly self-righteous feelings of superiority which the nondisabled have displayed toward persons with disabilities for centuries.

There is evidence of a growing rift between disabled citizens and professionals in rehabilitation as well as other fields. I have recently learned that the Royal Association of Disability and Rehabilitation (RADAR) has adopted a position in opposition to the passage of antidiscrimination legislation in the United Kingdom. This stand is antithetical to the views of British leaders of organizations of disabled persons whom I have quoted in this analysis. RADAR's position may be consistent with the traditional understanding which regards improvements in functional and occupational skills as the sole solution to the problems confronting disabled people. But this could be an enormously short-sighted and foolhardy posture. Unless rehabilitation personnel become actively involved in supporting efforts by the disability rights movement to eliminate environmental and attitudinal bias and discrimination, there is a grave risk of increasing separation between disabled citizens and nondisabled professionals. The consequences could be detrimental to both groups. Without the services provided by rehabilitation and other professionals, disabled individuals might be deprived of an important resource in an environment which is not yet adapted to their needs and wishes. But without the tacit support of disabled citizens, the political credibility of rehabilitation leaders would be seriously undermined.

This schism is beginning to develop in the academic community. Many disabled scholars in the the United States are beginning to argue that they have not been adequately involved in decisions about research priorities and support. They do not feel they have received a proportionate share of the resources available from government agencies and foundations especially in rehabilitation and other disability-related disciplines. Some point out that an institute created to study the problems facing women would not be expected to grant most of its funds to males, but the support provided by similar centers for research on disability and rehabilitation has been disproportionately awarded to the nondisabled. Part of the problem extends beyond the usual obstacles which confront minority groups in academic life. Increasingly, disabled professors have expressed dissatisfaction with the theories and values which have dominated the study of disability in fields such as psychology, sociology, history, social work, education, architecture, law, and other areas.

They too are engaged in a struggle to alter theoretical frameworks so that increased attention can be focused on what they consider the most critical problems encountered by people with disabilities. Many are forming an organization known as the Disability Forum to promote the allocation of resources to disabled researchers and to develop proposals which might contribute to significant changes in policy and research on disability. Until nondisabled professionals are willing to cooperate with disabled persons in the attainment of these goals, research on disability may reflect the competing paradigms outlined here.

These comments should not be interpreted to mean that I regard established rehabilitation perspectives and the new approach based on concepts of equality and civil rights to be polar opposites doomed to exist side by side with little, if any, relationship to each other. On the contrary, I expect increasing numbers of rehabilitation professionals to embrace the alternative paradigm which I have proposed. Perhaps other analysts will find a means of reconciling these models or a method of incorporating the socio-political approach into the existing theoretical framework of rehabilitation. Although the task seems to require more wisdom than I possess, I would certainly applaud efforts in this direction. Meanwhile, I can only ascribe the disagreement between Croxen and me to the basic tension between these paradigms and to fundamental differences in social values. Perhaps the conflict also relates to the different experiences of disabled and nondisabled persons. Some might not prefer to acknowledge this possibility, but I find it difficult to deny that continuing involvement with a disability could have contributed to this result.

I can only hope that this debate will have at least one salutary effect. I trust that it will focus increased attention on the ideas contained in this analysis. Some readers may conclude that they support Croxen's sweeping condemnation of my work. A few might agree with me. Others may find special merit in some of the thoughts expressed by either side. However, I would implore readers to evaluate the ideas carefully before reaching a final judgment. In addition, I hope that further research will be conducted on quotas and other provisions of disability policy as well as the emerging international social and political movement of disabled citizens. I believe that the field of rehabilitation is ready to consider fresh, original, and creative concepts. I also feel that much of this future research must be performed by scholars who are personally familiar with the major principles of the disability rights movement. Without a constructive dialogue between representatives of this movement and rehabilitation professionals, both groups could suffer irreparable harm.

The intensity of this exchange seems to demonstrate once again that important changes seldom occur in the absence of conflict. Thoughts that imply significant challenges to established theories and practices eventually must be tested in the market place of ideas.

MONOGRAPHS IN THE SERIES'

Project Year 1978-80

#1 Readaptation After myocardial Infarction
Harold Sanne, M.D.
Goteborg, Sweden

#2 Hospital Based Community Support
Services for Recovering Chronic Schizophrenics:
The Experience at Lillhagen Hospital, Goteborg,
Sweden
Sven-Jonas Dencker, M.D.
Lillhagen Hospital
Sweden

#3 Vocational Training for Independent Living
Trevor R. Parmenter, B.A.
Macquarie University
Australia

#4 The Value of Independent Living: Looking at
Cost Effectiveness in the U.K. (Issues for
Discussion in the U.S.)
Jean Simkins
The Economist Intelligence Unit
London, England

#5 Attitudes and Disabled People: Issues for
Discussion
Vic Finkelstein, B.A.
The Open University
Great Britain

#6 Early Rehabilitation at the Work Place
Aila Jarvikoski
Rehabilitation Foundation
Helsinki

#7 The Role of Special Education in an Overall
Rehabilitation Program
Birgit Dyssegaard
Denmark

Project Year 1980-81

#8 Justice, Liberty, Compassion: Analysis of
and Implications for ''Humane'' Health Care and
Rehabilitation in the U.S. (Some Lessons from
Sweden)
Ruth Purtilo, Ph.D.
U.S.

#9 Rehabilitation Medicine: The State of the
Art
Alex Chantraine, M.D.
Switzerland

#10 Interchange of American and European
Concepts of Independent Living and Consumer
Involvement of and by Disabled People
Gini Laurie
Editor, Rehabilitation Gazette
and
Lex and Joyce Frieden
Houston, Texas

#11 The Prevention of Pressure Sores for
Persons with Spinal Cord Injuries
Philip C. Noble
Royal Perth Hospital
Australia

#12 Systems of Information in Disability and
Rehabilitation
Dr. Philip H.N. Wood
U.K.

#13 Verbotonal Method for Rehabilitation
People with Communication Problems
Dr. Carl Asp
University of Tennessee
and
Dr. Petar Gurbina
Yugoslavia

Project Year 1981-82

#14 Childhood Disability in the Family
Dr. Elizabeth Zucman
France

#15 A National Transport System for Severely
Disabled Persons—A Swedish Model
Birger Roos
Sweden

#16 The Clinical Attitude in Rehabilitation: A
Cross-Cultural View
Joseph Stubbins, Ph.D.
U.S.

#17 Information Systems on Technical Aids for
the Disabled
James F. Garrett, Ph.D., Editor
U.S. (WRF)

Project Year 1982-83

#18 International Approaches to Issues in
Pulmonary Disease
Irving Kass, M.D., Editor
U.S.

#19 Australian Approaches to Rehabilitation in
Neurotrauma and Spinal Cord Injury
James F. Garrett, Ph.D., Editor
U.S. (WRF)

#20 Work Site Adaptations for Workers with
Disabilities: A Handbook from Sweden
Gerd Elmfeldt, et al.
Sweden

#21 Rehabilitation in Australia: U.S.
Observation
Diane E. Woods, Editor
U.S. (WRF)

#23 Methods of Improving Verbal and Psychological Development in Children with Cerebral Palsy in the Soviet Union
L.A. Danilova
USSR

Project Year 1983-84

#24 Language Rehabilitation After Stroke: A Linguistic Model
Dr. Gunther Peuser
Federal Republic of Germany

#25 Societal Provision for the Long-Term Needs of the Mentally and Physically Disabled in Britain and in Sweden Relative to Decision-Making in Newborn Intensive Care Units
Ernle W.D. Young, Ph.D.
U.S.

#26 Community-Based Rehabilitation Services: The Experience of Bacolod, Philippines and the Asia/Pacific Region
Dr. Antonio O. Periquet
The Philippines

#27 Three Models of Independent Living in the Netherlands
Gerben DeJong, Ph.D.
U.S.

#28 The Future of Work and Disabled Persons
Paul Cornes
U.K.
and
Harlan Hahn, Ph.D.
U.S.

#29 Issues of Equality: European Perceptions of Employment Policy and Disabled Persons
Harlan Hahn, Ph.D.

*The Clinical Model in Rehabilitation and Alternatives (13 commentaries on monograph #16)

The following monographs are still available (*or will be*) in limited supplies: #12, #14, #15, #17, #18, #20, #21, #24-29, *.

INTERNATIONAL EXCHANGE OF EXPERTS AND INFORMATION IN REHABILITATION

WORLD REHABILITATION FUND, INC.
400 East 34th Street
New York, NY 10016

Howard A. Rusk, M.D.,
  Chairman of the Board

Howard A. Rusk, Jr.
  President
James F. Garrett, Ph.D.,
  *Executive Vice President,
  and Principal Investigator*

Diane E. Woods,
  Project Director

Theresa Brown,
  Project Secretary

Sylvia Wackstein,
  Secretary-Treasurer, WRF

INTERNATIONAL ADVISORY COUNCIL

Luis Vales Ancoma, M.D.
  Mexico
Diane de Castellane
  Paris, France
Professor Olle Hook, M.D.
  Goteborg, Sweden
Kurt-Alfons Jochheim, M.D.
  Federal Republic of
  Germany
Dr. Birgit Dyssegaard
  Denmark

Barbara Keller
  Zurich, Switzerland
Yoko Kojima, Ph.D.,
  Professor
  Tokyo, Japan
Douglas Limberick
  Australia
Armand Maron, Ph.D.
  Belgium
Seppo Matinvesi
  Finland

Sulejman Masovic
  Zagreb, Yugoslavia
C.W. de Ruijter
  Hoensbroek, Netherlands
Jack Sarney
  Canada
Teesa Selli Serra
  Rome, Italy
George Wilson
  London, England

INTERNATIONAL EXCHANGE OF EXPERTS
AND INFORMATION IN REHABILITATION

PEER REVIEW UTILIZATION PANEL
(U.S. ADVISORY COUNCIL)

Sheila Akabas, Ph.D.
Director
  Industrial Social Welfare
  Center
  The Columbia University
  School of Social Work
Thomas P. Anderson, M.D.
  Department of Physical
  Medicine and
  Rehabilitation
  University of Minnesota

Donn Brolin, Ph.D.,
  Professor
  University of
  Missouri-Columbia
Richard E. Desmond, Ph.D.
  Chairman
  Department of Special
  Education &
  Rehabilitation

Ruth R. Green,
  Administrator
  N.Y. League for the
  Hard of Hearing
Gini Laurie
  Rehabilitation Gazette
Kenneth Mitchell, Ph.D.
  Private Consultant
  to Industry

Mark Fuhrer, Ph.D.
  Texas Institute for
  Rehabilitation
  and Research
Claude A. Myer, Director
  Division of Vocational
  Rehabilitation Services

Carolyn Vash, Ph.D
Planning Systems
International, Inc.

SPECIAL CONSULTANTS TO PROJECT:

Leonard Diller, Ph.D.
  Institute of
  Rehabilitation Medicine
  NYU Medical Center

John Muthard, Ph.D.
  Rehabilitation
  Research Institute
  University of Florida

COOPERATING INTERNATIONAL ORGANIZATIONS
(U.S. Based)

University Centers for
International Rehabilitation
  William D. Frye, Ph.D.,
  Director, Michigan State
  University, Michigan

Rehabilitation International
U.S.A.
  Philip Puleio, Ph.D.,
  New York
Rehabilitation International
  Norman Acton, Secretary
  General, New York

Partners of the Americas
Gregg Dixon,
Washington, DC